Tribal Ethnomedicine : Continuity and Change

Tribal Ethnomedicine : Continuity and Change

by

JOSE BOBAN. K.

A.P.H. PUBLISHING CORPORATION
5, ANSARI ROAD, DARYA GANJ
NEW DELHI - 110 002

Published by
S.B. Nangia
A P H Publishing Corporation
4435-36/7, Ansari Road, Daryaganj
New Delhi 110002
Ph.: 23274050
E-mail : aphbooks@gmail.com

ISBN 81-7648-027-4

2023

Printed at
Balaji Offset
Navin Shahdara, Delhi 110032

Dedicated
to
my
Beloved
Parents

Preface

Through this book I attempt to present before you one of the little explored aspects of tribal life. In our country a large number of tribal studies are published every year. But these works mainly deal with some popular aspects of tribal culture like religion, family, kinship, folklore, cultural change, problems of development, etc. They generally give only scant attention to the health problems and medical practices of tribals. Actually, the tribals themselves are very concerned about the emerging health problems in their communities. Especially after their prolonged contact with non-tribals, many new diseases have become common among them. Their traditional medicinemen are unable to deal with these new ailments.

On the other hand the government is implementing so many health programmes for the tribals. On many occasions these efforts are not very successful, as the tribals do not come forward to avail of the benefits of such programmes. Moreover the medical personnel are also not happy working in tribal areas and hence the communication between these two groups is generally very poor. Additionally, these professionals are not able to understand the view-point of tribals. Very often they do not know that tribals themselves have a well developed ethnomedical system as a part of their culture. Therefore, through this study the author analyses this dilemma and suggests some solutions to overcome the mutual suspicion between the practitioners of modern medicine and tribals.

It is really amazing to notice that almost all aspects of tribal culture are influenced by religious beliefs. Even though their religion is not well organized like that of the non-tribals, they are very pragmatic in their attitude towards the supernatural. The influence of religion on ethnomedicine is very direct and profound, and even the basic principles of ethnomedicine are derived from religious concepts. This study has taken all pains to explain the complex connections between ethnomedicine and various aspects of tribal life, like religion, life cycle, world-view, rituals, occupation, level of acculturation, extent of isolation from non-tribals, etc. I hope that the planners, administrators, social workers, medical practitioners and all others concerned with the welfare of the tribals will find this book useful.

Fond memories of my association with the tribals will always remain with me. Their semi-isolated life inside the woods helps them preserve many of the natural, endearing human qualities even today. This book would not have seen the light of day but for the cooperation of the tribal brethren of Idukki district.

I do not think it sentimental to extend my appreciation to my beloved parents whose love and support has been for me a lifelong inspiration. I am immensely indebted to my nephew Augustine who helped me a lot during the fieldwork of the present study. I am really thankful to my wife for her wholehearted support in this project. The author also thanks S.B. Nangia of APH Publishing Corporation for bringing out this book in its present form.

JOSE BOBAN. K.

Acknowledgement

This is the outcome of my research on the Muthuvan and the Mannan Tribes residing in the Idukki District of Kerala State. An attempt has been made in this study to examine the ethnomedical practices found among the two tribes and the extent to which their system is influenced by various factors of change.

The study was carried out under the supervision and inspiring guidance of Dr. Jacob John Kattakayam, Reader in the Department of Sociology, University of Kerala. But for his scholarly guidance and encouragement, this study would not have been completed. I take this opportunity to place on record my gratitude and indebtedness to Dr. John for his valuable guidance, scholarly interest and singular attention shown throughout this study..

Dr. P.K.B. Nayar, Prof. and former Head, Department of Sociology, University of Kerala, extended to me very generous, and untiring help during the study. I acknowledge with thanks the keen interest and friendly encouragement he showed in my work.

My thanks are also due to the members of the Muthuvan and the Mannan communities. I always remember with gratitude their hospitality and cooperation extended to me during the course of my field work.

Fond memories of my association with the tribals will always remain with me. Their semi-isolated life inside the woods helps them preserve many of the natural, endearing human qualities even today. This book would not have seen the light of day but for the cooperation of the tribal brethren of Idukki district.

I do not think it sentimental to extend my appreciation to my beloved parents whose love and support has been for me a lifelong inspiration. I am immensely indebted to my nephew Augustine who helped me a lot during the fieldwork of the present study. I am really thankful to my wife for her wholehearted support in this project. The author also thanks S.B. Nangia of APH Publishing Corporation for bringing out this book in its present form.

In the end I would like to thank my fellow research scholars and friends who have been a source of great strength to me in my research work. I remember them all and my gratitude can find no adequate expression in words.

JOSE BOBAN. K.

CONTENTS

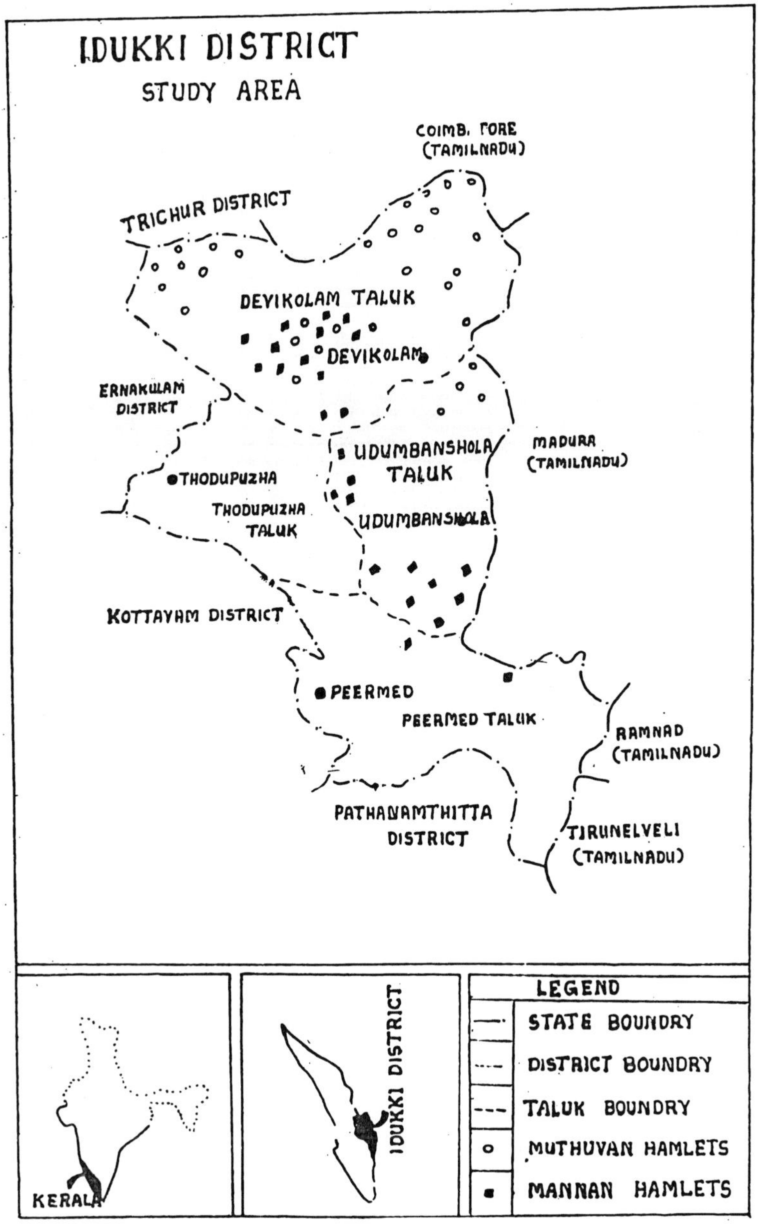
IDUKKI DISTRICT
STUDY AREA
COIMB. TORE
(TAMILNADU)
TRICHUR DISTRICT
DEVIKOLAM TALUK
DEVIKOLAM
ERNAKULAM DISTRICT
UDUMBANSHOLA TALUK
MADURA
(TAMILNADU)
THODUPUZHA
THODUPUZHA TALUK
UDUMBANSHOLA
KOTTAYAM DISTRICT
PEERMED
PEERMED TALUK
RAMNAD
(TAMILNADU)
PATHANAMTHITTA DISTRICT
TIRUNELVELI
(TAMILNADU)
KERALA
IDUKKI DISTRICT
LEGEND
STATE BOUNDRY
DISTRICT BOUNDRY
TALUK BOUNDRY
MUTHUVAN HAMLETS
MANNAN HAMLETS

Map

1

Introduction

The objective of this book is to examine the medical practices and healing rituals existing in the tribal communities and to evaluate the changes occurring in the traditional medical system as a result of the influence of modern medicine. Most of the tribal communities, as a rule, live inside dense forests in hilly areas and consequently enjoy an effective isolation from the mainstream of the country. Their more or less isolated life prevents them from exploiting many of the advantages of modern civilization. On many occasions they are found rejecting the programmes of modernization implemented by the governmental and voluntary agencies. They are still depending upon their own traditional medical practices when contracted by diseases. The ingredients of their medicines include herbs in toto, roots, barks, leaves, fruits and other plant parts, animal derivatives and also a few minerals. They have certain age-old techniques and methods of preparation and administration of medicines for different diseases. Healing rituals employed for invoking the intervention of supernatural forces, are an integral component of the treatment procedure. On the whole, it seems that traditional medicine helps the tribals to check the diseases satisfactorily and to lead a healthy life.

However, ethnomedicine of the tribals is now influenced by a number of forces external to the community, which are capable of bringing out changes into this traditional system. Modern medicine is the most important agent of change influencing the ethnomedical system. As a part of the tribal welfare programmes, the government has opened a number of curative centres like hospitals, dispensaries and Primary Health Centres (PHC) in the tribal areas and also has employed mobile dispensaries to improve the availability of medical facilities for them. In addition to this modern medicine is also available to them from a number of private nursing homes and hospitals, functioning in rural areas within an easily reachable distance from the abode of the tribals. However, on many occasions, the tribals show much reluctance in accepting modern medicine, for the treatment of diseases. It is observed that sometimes their resistance towards modern medicine is disease specific. They accept modern medicine for certain diseases, but reject it for some others. This selective approach is a major hurdle for the health personnel in the successful implementation of their programmes, and is also an interesting topic for social anthropologists to deal with.

Hence, the problem proposed to be investigated in the present study is the ethnomedical practices found among the tribals and the extent to which this system is influenced by various factors of change. The problem has two major and equally important aspects. The first aspect is a descriptive study of the traditional ethnomedical practices which are instrumental in the diagnosis, healing and prevention of various diseases and its inner ramifications with other aspects of tribal life, like social organization, religion, life cycle, etc. The second aspect of the problem deals with the challenges of medical pluralism upon ethnomedicine and the ways in which this system manages to survive (even though in a subdued manner) in a period of general social change which is occurring as a result of various tribal welfare measures of the government and also with increased interaction with the nontribals.

RELEVANCE OF THE STUDY

Study of the medical systems of tribal communities and their health problems is very relevant in view of acquiring knowledge of the health care practices of this section of population and also such information carry obvious policy and planning implications as well. These types of studies can point out the pit-falls inherent in the policies and programmes for tribal health care and can suggest remedies for rectifying these drawbacks. The scarcity of the number of studies dealing with this problem is a great impediment for the planners and policy makers to assess the existing situation among the tribal communities. According to Chaudhuri: " .... data on tribal health, concept of disease and nature of treatment are rather scanty and specific study on this topic with reference to the tribals covering the different facets is practically non-existent" (1986:5).

The study of the health problems needs special attention in the context of the tribal communities of India. Firstly, most of the Indian tribes are very backward with little social and material development and are living in isolated or remote areas where modern health facilities are not available. Secondly, it is observed that in some tribal communities, the mortality and morbidity rates are rather high in comparison to the corresponding rates of the general population of the country. Studies illuminating the health problems and medical practices existing in those tribal communities, can provide answers whether the current health care practices followed in those communities are responsible for such a situation.

The government is implementing a number of programmes for raising the standard of health of the tribals. However, it is observed that such programmes are not often successful in delivering good results. The medical practitioners and public health workers belonging to different parts of India have been reporting that very often the tribals do not utilize the medical, preventive and family planning facilities available to them. This is an important dilemma for the health planners and medical practitioners of our country. The solution to this intricate problem can be reached only through a systematic study of the tribal concepts of etiology, treatment of diseases and the role of a physician in the curing procedure. Such studies can prove whether dependence and confidence on tribal medicinemen and shamans are responsible for the non-acceptance of modern medicine, as ethnomedicine establishes faith and assurance in the patients, while the modern medicine lacks this aura of conviction'. Unless and until the reasons of failure are brought to light, the very health care programmes for the tribals cannot be successful.

The failure of health programmes can also be attributed to the fact that, as a large number of tribal communities are of varied socio-cultural traditions, economy and level of acculturation, their concepts of disease and methods of treatment are likely to be different. The results obtained through systematic study of the health care concepts of these different tribal communities will be helpful for the planners and policy makers to formulate suitable plans for each community. Hasan has opined that success in public health programmes often depends upon modifications in human behaviour. He further explained it as follows: "The process of planning, organizing and operating the medical and health programmes, therefore, demands that the persons entrusted with such tasks should have a knowledge of the general concepts of culture and social organization and a thorough understanding of various social institutions of the community in which the programme is to be carried out" (1967:2).

In order to avoid misunderstandings between a doctor and his patients it is recommended that a good working knowledge of the tribals' own concepts of etiology of illness, methods of treatment and their expectations of the role of a physician can enable a doctor to behave in the appropriate manner. The dearth of studies dealing with the tribal concepts of etiology and curing is a major handicap for such physicians and health-workers who want to enlighten themselves of these information. To cite another example, it is a generally accepted fact that no progress in environmental sanitation is possible without proper health education. But the basic problem with the health administrators is 'what to educate? and how to educate? No relevant data on the sanitary habits of the tribals are available for understanding the present situation. Without understanding the sanitary practices existing among the tribals at present, how can the health educators ask these people to adopt new healthy habits.

Supernatural beliefs and healing rituals occupy a prominent place in the treatment of diseases like epilepsy, chest pain, measles, successive abortions, insanity, etc., which are supposed to have originated from supernatural causes. Tribals have much reluctance to accept modern medicine for the treatment of such supernatural diseases as they believe that no material medicine is efficacious in checking them. On the other hand, they resort to invoke the assistance of supernatural forces on such occasions. While implementing the health programmes, proper consideration of such cultural inhibitions is necessary to avoid friction and misunderstanding between the tribals and the practitioners of modern medicine.

A number of medicines used by the tribals may be potentially effective in the treatment of various diseases. A team of experts comprising of botanists, taxonomists, chemists, druggists and anthropologists can collect the various plant, animal and mineral substances used by the tribals for preparing their medicines. Then, by scientific analysis of these materials a number of efficacious medicines can be invented from them. Primarily social scientists can invite the attention of these experts by recording the ethnomedical practices of different tribes in their studies and disseminate this information to the scientific community and also to the general public. Several scholars have highlighted the importance of tribal medicine in their studies (Mathur 1982, Nair 1985 Narayan 1986, Bhattacharjee et. al. 1986 and Joseph 1989) and complained about the present indifferent attitude of scientists, towards this system of medicine. After the introduction of modern medicine even some tribals underestimate the importance of their own ethnomedicine. So there is an urgent need to record the ethnomedical practices present among different tribal communities; particularly the use of herbal medicines should be documented before they are forgotten. A study of the traditional mode of contraception is also very important. The details about herbal contraceptives used by the tribals must be collected and through scientific experiments, a refined form of it can be produced for the use of the non-tribal population also. If such contraceptives have no side effects, then it will be a great boon for the family welfare programmes of the country.

SELECTION OF THE TRIBES

The Muthuvan and the Mannan are the two tribal communities selected for the present study. Both are hill tribes living in the mountaineous regions of the Idukki district of Kerala state (South India). Idukki district has, a tribal population of 3.98 percent of the total population. According to 1981 census the total number of the Muthuvan population is 11,213 and of the Mannans is 5,813.

Two tribal communities are selected in order to improve the reliability and authenticity of the study and to ensure that the generalizations drawn from the study are more accurate. It is generally accepted that the results obtained by an analysis of more qualitative as well as quantitative data will be more accurate. It is observed that each tribal community possesses its own unique culture, and each one's response towards the outside influences is different. So the study of different tribal communities will indicate the structural, ecological and cultural factors that determine their differential behaviour.

Even though the two tribal communities selected for the present study, viz., the Muthuvan and the Mannan inhabit the same district, they possess more differences than similarities. First of all they belong to different economic categories. The Muthuvans are shifting cultivators while the Mannans are settled agriculturalists. The difference in occupation is a signal of the differences in all other spheres of life.

The Muthuvans who follow the traditional occupation of shifting cultivation are very backward and majority of them live inside dense forests. The Muthuvan community is a closely knit body and the members have strong bonds of mutual attachment. The rigid social organization, group cohesion, mutual dependence, strong leadership and effective isolation from the modern civilization are the major reasons which help them to resist the outside influences and to preserve the purity of their culture.

'The Muthuvans consider themselves as superior to all other tribal and non-tribal societies and believe that their culture and mode of living are very appropriate to the environment in which they live. They show little affinity to imitate the non-tribal culture and do not like to mingle freely with the outsiders. They do not share cooked food with other tribal communities and observe pollution to certain communities like the Mannans, Hill Pulayas, Parayans and Chakkiliyans. Their womenfolk enjoy little freedom to mingle with the outsiders of the community.

The Muthuvans have no enthusiasm to avail the facilities provided by the government through various welfare programmes. This is one of the major reasons for their socio-economic backwardness. This indifference is manifest in the area of health care programmes also. Majority of them still wholly depend upon ethnomedicine for the treatment of diseases. They have an array of efficacious medicines which are capable of checking various diseases. A number of shamans possessing great knowledge in various magical spells and healing rituals are also present in the Muthuvan community. Therefore, the Muthuvans have all the resources to tackle the illnesses afflicting them and they do not believe that modern medicine is essential for them to preserve their health. As they are less exposed to modern medicine, they have only limited experience with the advantages of this medical system. This lack of familiarity often discourages them to seek the assistance of modern medicine when afflicted by diseases. However, a small minority living in the fringe areas of forests accept modern medicine more readily than their counterparts living in the interior areas. They are also very reserved like their brethren and accept modern medicine when afflicted by serious diseases only.

On the other hand the Mannans are entirely different from the Muthuvans in many respects. Most of the Mannan hamlets are located in the fringe areas of forests with a lot of connections with the nearby towns. In addition to the major occupation of settled agriculture, the Mannans go for manual labour also in the nearby plantations owned by the government and the non-tribals. Both men and women are employed as wage labourers in these plantations. These circumstances lead to more contacts with the outsiders of the community. As a result of close association with the non-tribals the Mannans imbibe a number of non-tribal features into their life.

The community rules and customs have become less rigid among the Mannans, after the contact with the modern civilization. Today the community tolerates the freedom of the individual members and the cohesion of the group is gradually dwindling. Their present leadership is very weak and is losing its authority over the community members. Even the authority of the headman of a hamlet is being challenged by the members in many places and very often he is only a nominal leader of the hamlet, with limited powers. So, the Mannans are becoming more individualistic, which adversely affect the cohesion of the community. Their womenfolk also enjoy much freedom and there is no custom which prevents them from mingling with the outsiders. The weakness of leadership and the existence of individual freedom enable the Mannans to accept the new innovations like modern medicine, which are brought by the government and other voluntary agencies.

It is observed that the Mannans generally cooperate with the welfare programmes of the government. This is true in the area of health care also. Traditionally the Mannans possess a well developed ethnomedical system, and there are a number of expert medicinemen and shamans in their community. They know how to treat various ailments with the assistance of herbal medicines and healing rituals. Still, the Mannans show very little resistance in accepting the modern medical facilities. As they are living in the fringe areas of forests, modern medicine is easily accessible to the Mannans, and they utilize such facilities in addition to their ethnomedicine. Thus, the Mannans are more exposed to the modern medical facilities, unlike the Muthuvans who live isolated inside the dense forests.

The Muthuvans and the Mannans were exposed to the foreign influences, more or less in the same manner. But each community responded towards these alien forces in quite different manner. When the non-tribal immigrants and government officials reached their abode, the Muthuvans retreated towards more interior areas of forests, in order to preserve the purity of their culture and traditions in that sylvan isolation. This withdrawal helped them to keep alive their ethnomedicine also which is an integral part of their culture. On the other hand, the response of the Mannans towards modern civilization was entirely different from that of the Muthuvans. Even though they have not readily accepted the modern culture in the early periods of contact; they have been very tolerant towards these alien influences. With the passage of time they have accepted certain aspects of modern civilization which they thought beneficial for them. This is manifest in their attitude towards medical practices also. Now they are pragmatically availing the modern as well as ethnomedical facilities according to the need of the circumstance.

In this way the Muthuvans and the Mannans show much different behaviour, when confronted with modern civilization. This is an interesting situation which invites thorough analysis in the anthropological line. The difference between the two tribes is reflected in their attitude towards modern medicine also. Through this study an attempt has been made to understand the ethnomedical system of the Muthuvans and the Mannans and the differences as well as similarities in their approach towards modern medicine. It is also investigated whether the cultural peculiarities of the Muthuvans and the Mannans are responsible for the differential acceptance of the modern health care practices. A study of these two tribal communities is very relevant because; the Muthuvans and the Mannans are two tribes having differential educational and acculturation status; they belong to different economic category and; the Mannans are well exposed to the modern medical facilities while the Muthuvans are less exposed to modern medicine due to their comparative isolation from the modern civilization.

MEDICINE AND SOCIETY

Every human society in the world, irrespective of its degree of cultural and material simplicity or complexity, has maintained an effective medical system and possessed empirically tested knowledge about etiology and curing, to cope with the diseases which threaten the well-being of its members. Very often, these traditional medical beliefs and practices may not appear quite rational, when viewed from the conceptual framework of modern scientific medicine. But it worked satisfactorily with the people who made use of it.

The success of a medical system can be evaluated by examining how the people utilizing this knowledge and its methods are maintaining their health and living in harmony with their environment. While going through the evolutionary history of mankind, one can find that the notion of health, disease and healing practices constitute an important part of the human culture itself. Diseases threatened man's existence on earth and human societies were forced to invent a pharmacopoeia and to develop therapeutic measures to win over the challenges from his environment.

The medical system in a society is related to all the other spheres of social life, and therefore medicine can be considered as a sub-system, regulated and influenced by the world view and material development of the wider social system. Social anthropologists have been very keen in exploring the patterns of interaction between the sub-system of medicine and the major system of society, which ultimately paved the way for the emergence of a new discipline in social sciences known as medical anthropology. This science deals with the complex connections between a folk therapeutic system and the culture within which it operates.

Fabriga has given a definition of medical anthropology as follows:

"A medical anthropology inquiry will be defined as one that (a) elucidates the factors, mechanisms and processes that play a role on or influence the way in which individuals and groups are affected by and respond to illness and disease and, (b) examines these problems with an emphasis on patterns of behaviour" (1972:189). According to him, neither concepts, methods nor aims are critical, but rather the content of the work that is performed. Thus, medical anthropology's major areas of concern, are, society's beliefs, concepts and curative measures of illness, and to explain how the people cope with a disease, and what solution they offer to overcome this situation, in the general background of their culture.

One cannot examine the medical system of a society in isolation, since the beliefs and practices related to disease, its causation and cure, are very much incorporated with so many other activities of a society. For understanding the medical beliefs and practices, one has to deal with almost all facets of social life, like the religious beliefs, rituals, values, norms, world view, interrelationship with other societies, material progress and the ecosystem in which the society is embedded. According to Lieban (1972 :1031) ".......... an anthropological study of health and the occurrence and means of coping with disease can involve one deeply in the manner in which people perceive their world, in the characteristics of human social systems, and in social values. In this perspective, medical anthropology is not only a way of viewing the states of health and disease in society, but a way of viewing society itself".

The tribals belong to the lowest class of the present day society and are showing only simple material development. The tribal societies are contemporary societies which more closely resemble communities of early man. Therefore, by the study of the diseases and medical systems of the tribals, one can attain more insight regarding the evolution of diseases in the human society. Polunin has stated, "Though contemporary tribal men cannot be equated with prehistoric men, they resemble them more than do modernized men. Therefore, the study of tribal peoples not only widens the range of circumstances in which human adaptability is observed. It throws some light on the evolution of human diseases" (1977:5).

It is noticeable that the tribals who are living in a harsh environment could manage to maintain good health and lead an active life with the help of their own medical practices and cultural etiquette. Their religious beliefs, cultural values and customs help them to regulate their activities and to exploit the resources from their environment without tilting its ecological balance. Their small groupsize and effective isolation from other human societies reduced the chances of being afflicted by most of the contagious diseases. The good health of the members of tribal societies is, however not a state characterized by the absence of disease but one of steady control at bearable levels.

Social anthropologists who have studied the primitive communities have shown great concern in studying their social organization, kinship, marriage, family, religion, economy, etc., while their medical beliefs and practices have been neglected. So the earlier monographs of many of the primitive communities often contain little narration in connection with disease and medicine. "It is true that all through the history of mankind attempts have been made to explain different aspects of medicine in terms of social variables. But it is only in the past fifty years or so that serious attempts have been made to study systematically the relation between the sub-culture of medicine and the wider society of which it is a part (Ahluwalia 1974 :401)

The study of the medical systems of tribal societies needs urgent attention, considering the influence of various agents which are inducing rapid changes in this section of the population. Most of the tribal societies are no longer enjoying complete isolation from other human groups and rapid social changes can be noticed due to the contact with the people of other cultures. Man induced changes like deforestation and monoculture afforestation altered their habitat and resulted in the non-availability of games, tubers, honey, medicinal herbs, fruits, etc. The various welfare measures of the government to raise the standard of life of the tribals accelerated the pace of these changes. Now, a number of tribes are following the life-style of the nontribal societies and their traditional norms, values, social institutions, and subsistence pattern have undergone vital transformation. So steps must be taken to study the ethnomedical practices of the tribals and to record all the efficacious medicines used by them, before they are lost.

The acculturation process has great influence on their health. Due to the close association with the members of other societies, they are now exposed to a number of new diseases which were not present among them earlier. Now a days many of the tribes are consuming food items available from ration shops and hotels. This new diet is very poor in quality when compared with the traditional type obtained from the forest. So, these changes have been detrimental to their nutrition and health.

More studies have to be conducted to understand the medical system of the tribals, the process of interaction between tribal medicine and modern medicine, and how both can cooperate to develop a health care system desirable for the tribals. Special emphasis must be given in these studies on sanitary facilities and the relevance of proper health education. The data available from such studies will be very useful in planning modern health services suited to tribal areas.

TRIBAL STUDIES IN KERALA

According to 1991 census, the Scheduled Tribe population of Kerala state is 320967 which works out to 1.10 percent of the total population. For India as a whole the percentage of Scheduled Tribe population is 7.8 during this period. The census of 1991 gives a list of 35 tribal communities in Kerala. Even though, the percentage of tribal population in Kerala is very negligible, considerable number of ethnographic works have been carried out here right from the last decades of the nineteenth century.

Earlier information about these tribes was brought to light in the descriptive notes of administrators, census officers and missionaries who worked here during the British rule. Abbe Dubois (1897) who was a French missionary, in his book, 'Hindu Manners, Customs and Ceremonies', gives an account of some wild tribes like, *Kadu Kurumbar, Irular, Malaikondigaru and Yeruvaru* of the Wayanad region. He described these people as savages.

Among the earlier administrators who had an interest on tribals, the name of Edgar Thurston figures prominently. He published the 'Ethnographic notes in Southern India, (1906) as well as seven volumes on 'Castes and Tribes of Southern India' (1909). In this series of seven volumes, Thurston gives a brief account of all the tribes and castes living in South India, arranged alphabetically. In his first book Thurston has described the several customs related to marriage, death, slavery, sacrifices, infanticide and couvad practised by the people of South India.

L.K. Anantakrishna Iyer undertook an ethnographic survey of the hill tribes and the low caste people of Cochin in South India. As a result of this investigation he published a book, 'Tribes and Castes of Cochin' (1908) in four volumes. His well arranged description covers the traditions, origin, ceremonial rites, religious beliefs and occupation of the tribal and fishing communities.

L.A. Krishna Iyer undertook the ethnographic survey of the primitive tribes and low castes of Travancore, South India in 1933. Iyer first concentrated on the hill tribes which were fast dying out or were getting assimilated into the tribes and castes of the plains. As a result of this study he wrote a book, 'The Travancore Tribes and Castes' in three volumes. The first volume (1937) contains an ethnographic account of seven hill tribes. The second (1939) and the third (1941) volumes of this book contain the descriptive accounts of the tribes of Travancore, and also the anthropometric and serological information about them. In another study (1961) he described the hill tribes of Kerala as 'Pre-Dravidians.' He also wrote an analytical paper on taboos among the tribes of Travancore. In a later study (1963) he put forward the opinion that there has been a peaceful penetration of the lower aboriginal culture by the higher Dravidians, and that the megaliths in South India are Pre-Dravidian in origin.

M.D. Raghavan did some field researches among the *Jain Kurumbas* of Travancore as early as 1929, the result of which has been published in 'Man in India' (1929) as a lengthy paper.

A.A.D. Luiz (1962) described the customs and ways of life of 48 tribes of Kerala in his book, 'Tribes of Kerala'. In his description he has recorded the details about the origin and growth of the tribes, their social structure, religious beliefs and rituals, material culture and marriage and death ceremonies.

Various scholars like Gnanambal (1955), Nag (1954), Ray (1955) and Mukherjee (1956) of Anthropological Survey of India studied the tribal communities of Kerala, especially the *Kanikkar*, the *Uraly* and the *Muthuvan* of Travancore. These studies are conducted from the religious, social-structural, demographic and psychological points of view.

Sengupta and Biswas conducted a dietary and nutritional survey among the *Malapantaram*, the *Muthuvan*, and the *Ullatan* tribes of Travancore and published a paper in the Bulletin of the Anthropological Survey of India (1956).

U.R. Ehrenfels (1952) studied the primitive *Kadar* tribe of Kerala and published a book, namely 'Kadars of Cochin'. This Monograph deals with the various aspects of Kadar culture and also brings out the changes that have taken place among the indigenous Kadar culture.

P.T. Harmanns (1955) published a paper on 'Kadar Religion' after a fieldwork among the *Kadars* living in the border district of Travancore Cochin.

Another scholar A. Aiyappan made a systematic study of the *Nayadis* of Malabar (1937).

P.T. Thomas (1952) made a sociological analysis of the political affiliation of the *Muthuvans* of Travancore. The religious beliefs and practices of the Muthuvans also have been studied by Thomas (1954) and published under the title 'Some observation on the religion of the Muthuvans'. In a later study (1963) he discussed, how an extra conservative tribe like the Muthuvans have made adjustments to the general changes in their environment. He clearly showed how organizational and occupational adjustments do occur among a primitive group confronted with the dynamism of modern developments and the influx of alien peoples.

P.R.G. Mathur (1977) divided the tribal communities of Kerala into seven major territorial groups taking into account their historical, ethnic, socio-cultural and religious background. He also studied the ethnomedical practices of the tribals of Wayanad (1982).

Jacob John Kattakayam (1983) conducted a study among the *Uralis* of Idukki and described their social structure, family life, economic organization, religion and social change in his book, 'Social Structure and Change among the Tribals'. He examined the failure of various governmental welfare programmes and suggested the measures to be taken to make these programmes effective and to ameliorate the lot of the tribals.

N. Viswanathan Nair (1985) undertook a research work about the tribal health and medicine in Kerala. He collected primary data from five tribal communities belonging to different modes of subsistence. This authentic and descriptive study dealing with ethnomedicine of tribals is one of the pioneering studies in the branch of medical anthropology in Kerala.

K. Mohandas (1987) conducted a study about the culture change and physical characteristics of *Paliyans* of Kerala. After describing their traditional customs and practices, he showed how these tribal features are transformed due to culture change.

The present review highlights the rich tradition of tribal studies in Kerala. Many of these studies provide much useful data about their culture, tradition, family, religion, social structure, ethnomedicine, social change, etc. However, it is noticeable that the research work in this field has not exhausted all the tribals and there are still a large number of tribal communities which are not studied by any anthropologist. Every tribal group has its own peculiarities and each one of them is undergoing rapid change. In order to make valid and reliable generalizations, they have to be based on the data collected from as many studies as possible. These are only a few among the large number of justifications which amply support the need for more studies of tribal communities.

HEALTH AND MEDICINE IN INDIA - A REVIEW

A study of medical systems and health is very interesting in the Indian context, because this country possesses an immense heterogeneity in medical beliefs and practices. Besides, the well known and wide spread medical systems such as Ayurveda, Allopathy, Unani and Homeopathy, there are various types of localized folk and tribal medical beliefs and practices often based on magic and sorcery. Since five decades or so there is no dearth of medical anthropological research in India. These studies mainly focused their attention on both tribal and less developed rural communities. Besides a description of their beliefs and practices about illness and medicine, the interaction between modern and traditional medical systems also forms an important aspect of these studies. Naik (1972) and Ahluwalia (1974) made useful surveys about the medical anthropological literature available in India which deals with the Indian tribal and rural communities.

TRIBAL HEALTH AND MEDICINE

Even the descriptive ethnographic literature compiled by the British administrators and missionaries did not fail to notice the primitive medical beliefs and practices found among the tribals. Since the diseases often threatened the existence of early tribal communities the concepts of etiology and curing methods had an important place in their culture.

Thurston (1907) described the beliefs in connection with charms, magical spells, witchcraft and sorcery for curing diseases and protecting people from evil spirits.

While discussing the religious belief of the Travancore tribes Krishna Iyer (1941) mentioned briefly about their medicineman who cures all their ailments and is a practitioner of magic. He says that propitiation of gods is intended to restore man's confidence when shaken by crises like accidents and diseases.

Sengupta and Biswas (1956) conducted a dietary and nutritional survey among the *Malapantaram*, the *Muthuvan* and Ullatan tribes of Travancore and made a comparison of the differences in the quality of their diet and its influence on their health and physical growth.

With a description of the disease causing spirits, taboos and the initiation and functions of the medicineman of the *Uralis*, Gnanambal (1955) also noticed that the Uralis make a fine distinction between the diseases of pathological origin and those of spirit origin.

Majumdar (1961) puts forward the opinion that social and cultural factors do play a major role in the spread of a disease.

Troisi (1979) made a fine analysis of the magic and witchcraft beliefs of the *Santals* of Bihar. He says that the *Santals* look upon most of the diseases as something unnatural, ascribing them to the agency of evil spirits and malevolent forces, witches and the evil eye.

Hockings (1980) presented an elaborate account of the indigenous medical system of the *Badagas* of South-India. He showed that their understanding of human physiology is rudimentary and misinformed.

Singh (1984) examined the drawbacks in the health policies of the government and the shortcomings in their implementation among the tribal communities. He points out that the government hospitals in the tribal areas are handicapped due to lack of equipment, medicine, and well motivated staff.

In a monograph of the War Khasis, a tribal community of Meghalaya, Dasgupta (1984) gives the impression that they are using both indigenous herbal medicines and modern allopathic medicines for the treatment of diseases. The influence of Christianity and education minimized the belief in spirits as the causative agents of diseases.

Egnor (1984) discussed how some healers in Madras established a special relationship with the deities and function as the vehicle of their power. It is found that during the healing sessions the deity will speak through the servant to each patient and the supernatural power acting through the healer will cure the illnesses.

Vidyarthi and Rai (1977) explained the belief of different tribals like *Ho, Jaintia, Korwa, Maler and Oraon* in malevolent spirits and powers which can cause diseases, famine, infertility and even death. These tribals also believe that there are some other spirits who protect the people from sickness and other misfortunes.

Mathur (1982, 1987) examined the etiology of illness, occurrence of diseases, curing techniques and the efficacy of ethnomedicine among the different tribal communities of Wayanad. He pointed out that their contact with the non-tribals had introduced new diseases and the spread of these diseases adversely affected the growth of their population.

Besides giving a brief description of the ethnomedical practices of the *Kanikkars* of Kerala, Radhakrishnan (1986) also showed that they know a large number of herbal medicaments for the treatment of various ailments.

In his study of the health and ethnomedicine of some tribes of Kerala, Viswanathan Nair (1985, 1987) gives much emphasis on how a tribal community's health is affected by the disturbances in the habitat and alien cultural contact. The study indicates that those tribal communities whose natural habitat remains relatively undisturbed use more herbal medicine than those whose habitats are disturbed.

Mahapatra (1986) found that the *Santals* of Bihar believe that the ultimate cause of disease and death is evil spirits and witches, and this belief influences their attitude towards life and community. They are convinced that the administration of medicine has to be supplemented by the practice of exorcism and divination.

Sen (1986) presented the demography, prevalence of illness, vices and health status of the *Andamanese*, which is one of the smallest tribal communities in this country. He also suggested effective measures to increase their fertility.

After examining the impact of three diseases, namely leprosy, malaria and tuberculosis which are more prevalent among the tribal communities in four blocks of West Bengal, Chowdhuri et. al. (1986) reached the conclusion that the tribals are quite ignorant of many of the diseases. The tribals are little aware of the importance of health and hygiene and the availability of modern medical facilities.

Guha (1986) presents a descriptive account of the folk medicine of the *Boro* tribe of Assam. After giving the details of the etiology, diagnosis, treatment and prophylactic measures of diseases, he makes an analysis of the impact of modern medicine upon the traditional one.

Bhattacharya and Sengupta (1986) observed that the general concept of disease among the *Birhor* hints at intra-social hostility and a high degree of insecurity owing to activities of the spirits. So they pay much importance to community cohesion and propitiation of spirits in order to prevent illnesses.

According to Dash (1986) the basic concept of illness among the *Paraja* of Orissa, is explained by magico-religious beliefs. However, besides the magico-religious treatment of the diseases, the herbal therapy is also very much prevalent among them.

Rizvi (1986) examined the health practices of the *Jaunsari* tribe of Uttar Pradesh and described their concept of etiology. As they believe that most of the diseases originate due to supernatural causes, they do not know or think that surroundings, hygiene and dietary habits may produce illnesses.

After conducting an empirical study among the *Kherwar*, the *Chero*, the *Kol*, the *Mar*, the *Oraon* and the *Munda* tribes of Bihar, Chakraborty (1986) found that these people prefer modern medicine because it brings speedy relief and is readily available. According to them ethnomedicine takes longer period to cure the patients and there is also scarcity of medicinal herbs.

Mukherjee (1986) carried out a research highlighting the gerentological problems in the *Ho*, the *Munda* and the *Sahtal* tribes of Bihar. He found that the health status of the aging members is more pathetic in acculturated hamlets than in the traditional ones.

After conducting an empirical study among the *Oraons* of Orissa, Sahu (1987) reached the conclusion that they are aware of the modern health services available in various institutions and make special efforts to avail these facilities when confronted with serious diseases.

In a case study of the *Asur*, the *Birgia* and the *Kisan* tribes of Bihar, Upadhyay (1987) showed how changes in their natural habitat due to deforestation brought adverse effect on their health. The tribal medicinemen fail to cure the new diseases which occurred due to causes like pollution, change of diet and close association with the non-tribals.

Reddy (1987) analysed the problems involved in the implementation of modern medicine among the tribal people. He suggested that a thorough knowledge of the indigenous medical beliefs and practices and the different cultural values attached to them has to be acquired and then the modern medicine has to be introduced in a phased manner side by side with the native medicines.

Tiwari (1987) studied the concepts of health and disease among the *Raj* and the *Shauka* tribes of Uttar Pradesh. He found that most of their illnesses derive from some of their age-old habits, poverty and the environment in which they live.

Bhowmik and Bagchi (1987) examined the health and nutritional aspects along with the frequency of diseases and treatment pattern of the *Lodha* and the *Mahali* tribes of West Bengal. They found that these tribals suffer from communicable diseases due to improper sanitation, lack of pure drinking water, open air defecation, etc.

In his study, Ramesh Menon (1988) explained how the tribes of Arunachal Pradesh attribute every disease or misfortune to a particular evil spirit. He found that patients suffering from psychosomatic ailments respond favourably to their shaman's treatment.

After conducting an ethnozoological survey among the thirty five tribal communities of Madhya Pradesh, Joseph (1989) brought out the role played by reptiles in tribal medicine. He found that the traditional medical system is economical and without any side effects.

RURAL HEALTH AND MEDICINE

The study of the health problems of the village folk attracted the attention of anthropologists, social workers and public health administrators, since very early times. The scarcity of pure drinking water, lack of sanitation facilities and malnutrition are only a few among the large number of hazards to the health of the villagers who form above 70 percent of the total population of India. Many of the health problems, concepts of etiology and curative techniques of the rural folk and tribals bear close resemblance. Therefore, a review of the literature of rural health and medicine will be much illuminative to understand the tribal health problems in a wider perspective.

Fuchs (1949) conducted a study of the common diseases affecting the *Nimar Balahis*, who are a group of scheduled caste people. He found that their socio-economic backwardness and unhygienic sanitary conditions are the major reasons for the occurrence of epidemics every year.

Carstairs (1955) studied the occurrence of diseases and the healing methods of the inhabitants of two villages in Rajasthan. From his own experiences with the villagers, he advises that the western medicine must be presented to the people in a way that will command conviction and acceptance. Again he (1983) explained how the villagers believe that diseases are caused by the activities of witches. He observed the changes taking place in a village community from 1950 to 1981 and found that the people show a stubborn resistance to change in the field of health care.

Marriott (1955) made an analysis of the various indigenous medical practices in the Kishan Garhi village of Uttar Pradesh and re-examined the role of the western doctor as it appears to the villagers in the context of their social organization and their own medical institutions. According to him, it would appear that if western medicine is to find a firm place in the village under present conditions its role must be defined according to village concepts and practices.

Gould (1957) noticed that among the different studies of culture change, very little material has been obtained from the zone of interaction between the so-called primitive and so-called scientific forms of medical practice as an aspect of the more general interaction between scientific and primitive technology. In another study he (1965) clearly identified the reasons for the villagers not wholeheartedly making use of the modern medical facilities available to them.

Khare (1959) argued that the failure of modern medicine in the folk communities is due to the ignorance of physicians about the beliefs and practices of people regarding illness and its treatment. In another study, he (1981) emphasized that the villager is adapting himself to the new system of medicine by firmly locating himself in the ethics of his own system and its cultural values.

Aiyappan (1965) made a few general observations on the health problems of the villagers and showed how the caste factor influences the doctor-patient relationship. He also explained how ecological factors like lack of sanitary conveniences, poor quality of drinking water and air pollution have led to the progressive deterioration of the health of the villagers.

Hasan (1967) presented an account of the beliefs, customs and practices of the village folk in relation to health and disease. He pointed out the weakness of modern medicine in the rural cultural context and suggested ways for the successful implementation of public health programmes.

According to Gorer (1967) the fear of illness and the ceremonies against it contributed, by far the largest impact of religion on the life of the *Lepchas*, a village community of Sikkim. In their view, the cause of all illnesses and misfortunes is the supernatural forces and, therefore, only supernatural methods are suitable for dealing with them.

Madan (1969) examined certain influences like rural or urban upbringing, age, education, occupation, income and religion of a person on his acceptance of modern medicine for himself and for planned change.

With a description of the concepts of etiology of some common diseases in a village, Karna

(1976) argued that the naturalistic interpretations of disease have more prominent place in the villager's concepts of etiology than the supernatural explanations.

Mandelbaum (1970, 1981) noticed that besides a number of purposes the villagers of India and Sri Lanka use their religion to restore the sick to health. He found that those ailments which could not be treated with drugs and techniques that are within the power of man, require the direct intervention of transhuman forces.

Djurfeldt and Lindberg (1976) made a detailed study of the health status and disease panorama of a Tamilnadu village. They found that the most fundamental reason for the apparent relative efficiency of indigenous medicine in the village is the inefficiency of the allopathic one.

Kakar (1977) made an exploratory study of the cultural context of certain diseases in a village in Panjab and offer helpful insight for further studies on health and nutrition in other villages.

Besides briefly discussing some aspects of ethnomedicine in Basanavahalli, a Karnataka village, Bhat (1976) revealed details of the circumstances and the forces that play a role in the initiation of a medicineman.

Matthews (1979) studied the effect of poverty on health in a South Indian village. She found that lack of proper understanding of the beliefs of the people and gaps in communication between the doctor and the patient have stood in the way of successful implementation of modern medicine.

Van Der Veen (1981) examined the various circumstances leading to the failure of a government sponsored Primary Health Centre (PHC) in a village. He found that the traditional village society could not wholly accommodate the technical medical concepts as well as an organization mainly based on western ideals and practices.

Mani (1981) studied the prevailing ethnomedical beliefs and practices regarding sterility, fertility, conception, gestation and abortion in rural Tamilnadu. He cautioned that any attempt at improving the health care system in rural India through the introduction of modern medical practices should be sensitive to the already existing complex network of ethnomedical beliefs and practices.

Henry (1981) studied the role and image of a North Indian magicoreligious medical practitioner and showed how he exploited the villagers' faith in his powers for healing. His mode of healing in which natural remedies are combined with exorcism, is an expression of a world view which comprehends both natural and supernatural causes of illness.

Nichter (1981) puts forward the view that the villagers' acceptance of modern medicine did not mean that they lost faith in their traditional medical system. Often, the use of allopathic medicine is constrained by cultural factors including indigenous notions of body physiology, etiology and diet.

Although it seems that modern medicine is accepted by a large number of rural people,

Bhardwaj (1985) cautioned that the increasing utilization of modern medicine does not mean that their attitude towards all aspects of modern curative and preventive medicine and family planning measures has undergone fundamental change.

CONCEPTS OF DISEASE ETIOLOGY

In tribal communities the concepts of etiology of disease can be broadly divided into two, natural causation and supernatural causation. In contrast to the nontribal societies where diseases are largely considered as natural phenomena which occur from a physiological malfunctioning of the body, the tribal communities give more importance to the supernatural causes in their notions of etiology. Therefore, cultural factors like religion, social status, relationship, with the fellow members of the society, nature of relationship with the supernatural world, etc., play a decisive role in the evolution of a concept of etiology in a tribal society.

Elwin (1955) studied the religious life, ethnomedicine, and culture of *Saora* tribe of Orissa. He said that the etiology of illness among the Saora tribe is based on supernatural beliefs. According to them all the diseases originated due to the wrath of the gods, dead ancestors and sorcerers. They identify no natural causes for the occurrence of diseases. Offering sacrifice to the supernatural and thus appeasing their anger is the only remedy for illnesses. The Saora theory of the origin of disease suggests that the gods and the dead ancestors have to make a living somehow and the only way they can do so is by forcing human beings to support them through sacrifices and other offerings. In many cases the only thing a Saora can say about a god is to name the disease he gives.

With respect to aetiological factors Saunder (1954) recognized three types of causation: empirical, magical and psychological. Empirical or 'natural' diseases are those in which a known external factor operates directly on the organism to produce the illness. Magical diseases are those in which the causative factors lie outside the realm of empirical knowledge and cannot be thus verified. Psychological diseases are those in which a strong emotional experience causes the appearance of the disease symptoms.

Simmons (1960) analysed the ethnomedical beliefs among the *Mestizo* communities in coastal Peru and Chile. Mestizo aetiological conceptions seek no support or sanction from religious or moral considerations, although a few are defined in supernatural terms. Consequently there is no single all-embracing causative factor such as incurring the displeasure of the benign or malevolent gods, that can provide a central integrated theory of disease. Instead, there are five major aetiological categories that embrace all of the serious illnesses and the vast majority of the minor ones. Illness is caused by severe emotional upset, contamination by ritually unclean persons, obstruction of the gastrointestinal tract, undue exposure to heat or cold, or exposure to 'mal air' or 'bad air'.

While giving an ethnographic account of disease causation and medicine in a tribal society,

Glick (1967) pointed out that whereas in Western medicine causation has no essential relationship to sociocultural context, in most other medical systems causation and context are so intimately linked as to be the ethnographer's principal concern. Causes may turn out to be as invisible as viruses, but never as impersonal. Causation has several dimensions, not all of equal importance. First, there is the relatively minor question of how an illness was brought about (instrumental cause); then there is the much more compelling question of who was the responsible agent (the efficient cause); and finally one encounters more extensive explanations of why the agents act as they do (ultimate cause), at which point one has moved beyond the realm of the medical system and into such considerations as social and political competition, intra-familial disputes, quarrels, conflicts and crimes.

Hughes (1968) in his well known article 'Ethnomedicine', illustrated the primitive concept of disease classification of Clements, in which there are-five basic categories of events or situations which in folk etiology, are believed responsible for illness: (1) sorcery, (2) breach of taboo, (3) intrusion of a disease object, (4) intrusion of a disease-causing spirit, and (5) loss of soul. He further elaborated that not every society recognizes all five categories; indeed many groups are selective in the emphasis placed upon one or a combination of causes.

Hughes has coined the term ethnomedicine, to denote the medical beliefs and practices found in primitive and folk societies, which is by and large accepted by anthropologists everywhere. He says: "The term ethnomedicine will be used to refer to those beliefs and practices relating to disease which are the products of indigenous cultural development and are not explicitly derived from the conceptual framework of modern medicine." (1968:88)

Foster (1976) in his account on disease etiologies in Non-Western medical systems identified two principal etiologies-personalistic and naturalistic. A personalistic medical system is one in which disease is explained as due to the 'active purposeful intervention' of an 'agent' who may be human, non-human or supernatural. In contrast to personalistic systems, naturalistic systems explain illness from such 'natural forces or conditions' as cold, heat, wind, dampness and above all, by an upset in the balance of the basic body elements.

Karna (1976) divided the concepts of etiology held by the dwellers of a Bihar village, into two categories, i.e. scientific concepts and conventional concepts. The disease causing agencies under scientific concepts are the external agents like mosquitoes and germs. The conventional concepts are further divided into natural and supernatural types of disease causation. The natural causes of disease include the quality of food, environmental conditions, personal habits, hardwork without adequate diet, and taking beef. Wrongs done to some god are the only cause that comes under the supernatural category of disease etiology.

After an exploratory study of the health culture of people in a North Indian village Hasan (1967) found that the village folk classified the causes of illness into two broad categories:

(1) supernatural and (2) physical. The supernatural causes of disease include (a) breach of taboo; (b) sorcery; (c) spirit intrusion; (d) evil eye; (e) wrath of gods and goddesses; and (f) ghost intrusion. The physical causes of illness recognized are (a) the effect of weather; (b) the effect of wrong food; (c) contact with certain living organisms; (d) blood getting impure; (e) accidents and natural calamities; and (f) unknown causes.

Murdock et.al. (1978) took a sample of 139 societies distributed fairly equally among the different geographical regions and classified their illness causation beliefs and theories. They are against the assumption that the primitive concepts of disease have little in common with those recognized by modern medical science and relate much more closely to the ideology of primitive religion.

The authors divided the illness causation beliefs into two, viz. the theories of natural causation and the theories of supernatural causation. The theories of natural causation account for the impairment of health as a physiological consequence of some experience of the victim in a manner that would not seem unreasonable to modern medical science. Infection, stress, organic deterioration, accident and overt human aggression are the five distinct types of theories which fall into the general category of theories of natural causation. Theories of supernatural causation rest on supernatural assumptions which modern medical science does not recognize as valid. They do, however, fall into three readily distinguishable groups, each of which is capable of separate definition: (1) theories of mystical causation, (2) theories of animistic causation, and (3) theories of magical causation. Theories of mystical causation are divided into four specific types of causation as fate, omnious sensations, contagion and mystical retribution. Theories of animistic causation are divided into two distinct types as soul loss and spirit aggression. Theories of magical causation are divided into two different categories as sorcery and witchcraft.

While giving an account of the traditional Iguape medical system, Queiroz (1984) said that in the analysis of any medical system the underlying notion of disease causation is crucial for determining diagnosis and treatment. The Iguape have three levels of causation for diseases. First, diseases can be caused by negative feelings from others (evil eye, sorcery) or from within oneself (sadness, unsatisfied will, fright). Secondly, they can be caused by an imbalance between the individual and his physical environment, as through the consumption of things considered too hot or too cold. Finally they can be caused by a deceased relative, by any evil spirit, even by the will of god. The first type of causation is social psychological, the second is natural and the third is supernatural.

Our review of literature reveals that the tribal communities are following a distinct way of life, entertain their own cultural values, possess viable mechanisms to adapt to their not so hospitable environment and have various techniques to cope with the diseases affecting them. The review also showed that almost all facets of tribal life are changing, due to contact with alien cultures and that the socio-political atmosphere of the country has accelerated this process of change.

Since the present study deals with ethnomedicine of tribals, it focuses attention on how ethnomedicine is influenced by modern medicine, and other agencies including the various welfare measures of the government.

One can come across with a voluminous account of tribal ethnography in India, dealing with various aspects of tribal culture. However, the number of studies giving due attention to the tribals, beliefs and practices related to disease, concepts of etiology and methods of treatment are very few in comparison with other aspects of tribal life, like religion, economy, kinship, marriage, etc. According to Glick "compared to the sophistication and organization of ethnographic accounts of social and political systems, even of religious systems, description of that body of beliefs and practices called 'medicine' lags far behind" (1967:52).

Even the existing studies are very sketchy and often with lots of gaps. So the present study will try to fill these lacunae and to contribute as much data as possible through the description of the ethnomedical system of the Muthuvans and the Mannans of Idukki district and examination of that system which is changing due to the influence of various agents. Such an analysis of ethnomedicine and medical pluralism will be very helpful in providing useful data for formulating relevant health care plans for tribal areas.

MEDICAL PLURALISM

One can notice that in many of the societies of the world people follow more than one type of medical system to deal with the illness situations. Even though the modern allopathic system is widely accepted in the world, many countries adopt their own traditional medical systems in addition to modern medicine. The Chinese Acupuncture and the Indian Ayurveda are only a few examples of this phenomenon which plays a complimentary role in the health care of the people, in the company of modern medicine. Practitioners of these diverse systems of medicine are following a give-and-take approach instead of an approach of contradiction and competition. Even though people are today making greater use of the modern medical facilities, they are also well aware of the importance of traditional medicine and prefer to take them for certain categories of illness. People have their own evaluations about the efficacy of the two systems of medicine for different illness. This selective use by the people help both systems of medicine to flourish in the same society.

Such a phenomenon of medical pluralism is very much alive in the case of tribal communities. In olden times the tribals who lived inside dense forests, completely isolated from the modern civilization, have been making use of their ethnomedicine for the treatment of whatever diseases afflicting them. But in the altered circumstances of the present day, the tribals are exposed to various kinds of medical systems in addition to their own. Even though they accept that modern medicine is efficacious in the treatment of various illnesses, they consider ethnomedicine as the only remedy for certain other illnesses. They cannot understand the logic of using modern medicine in illnesses caused by supernatural forces, but are ready to accept the efficacy of modern medicine in diseases occurring through natural causes. Thus they make an arbitrary division of the illnesses and use both systems of medicine selectively.

In a society where more than one system of medicine is operating one can notice their coexistence, instead of competition or contradiction. So the members of that society must be making suitable adaptations for the successful accommodation of the alien system. Young (1976) employed the concepts of 'assimilation' and 'particularization' to explain the phenomenon of medical pluralism where an alien medical system survives and functions successfully along with the traditional medical system of that society with an effective sharing of responsibilities regarding the health care of the people.

Young further explains this concept as follows: "Assimilation refers to instances where people utilize certain alien medical practices but, to the extent that they are knowledgeable about alien medical beliefs, they tend to assimilate these to homologous notions in their own medical system. Particularization occurs in three ways. (1) People believe that the alien medical system generates true etiologies, but that these etiologies can only account for 'new' sicknesses and not for any already incorporated into their folk system. (2) People believe that some of the practices of an alien system are effective, but only against (a) symptomatic complaints (since complete cures require the elimination of causal agents and only traditional measures are effective for this), or (b) a single category of symptomatically defined sickness. (3) People believe that another medical system generates etiologies that are empirically true, but they are relevant only to certain categories of people" (1976:10).

The concepts of assimilation and particularization thus successfully explain how tribals are looking upon the modern medicine which is an alien system for them. They seek modern medicine on many occasions and from the experiences which acquired through these interactions they have found that many of its therapies bring quick relief to certain maladies. Thus the people accept the efficacy of this new therapy and use them for the treatment of that particular category of diseases.

But it will be over enthusiastic to say that the tribals have accepted modern medicine 'wholeheartedly at the expense of their ethnomedicine. Actually they do not consider modern medicine as competent in treating many diseases including the ones caused by supernatural forces.

The tribals prefer to use the therapeutic measures of their ethnomedicine when afflicted with maladies which have been traditionally present in their community and they take modern medicine only for the newly imported diseases. They also believe that the modern medicine cures only the symptoms of disease and that the underlying causes can be eradicated only with the help of the shaman. So, even if the patient is undergoing treatment, the shaman must be approached to get a complete cure. It is a common practice that a patient who takes modern medicine also goes to the temple and makes offerings to god. Tribals believe that modern medicine is not efficacious in curing maladies like smallpox, measles, backache, jaundice, cholera and rheumatism, while they accept that it is effective in checking high fever, hernia, burns, pneumonia etc.

The term modern medicine is used in this study to denote all kinds of medical systems other than ethnomedicine, like allopathic, ayurvedic, homeopathic and unani systems of medicine. Among these different medical systems, generally allopathy alone could be considered as modern medicine. In the common usage ayurvedic, homeopathic and, unani systems of medicine are considered as traditional medicines. But in the context of the present study all systems of medicine except ethnomedicine are classified as modern, in order to draw a clear demarcation between the tribal and nontribal systems of medicine. The division of medical systems into modern and traditional is not much relevant for the tribals. In the past they were not in the habit of using any other systems of medicine whether traditional or allopathic. So, in their point of view, all the medical systems except their own are modern.

The phenomenon of medical pluralism is much relevant for the Muthuvans and the Mannans. Both the communities possess a well developed ethnomedical system. In addition to this, services of various other systems of medicine like allopathy, ayurveda and homeopathy are available to them as remedies for their diseases. The present study analyses the individual response of this two tribal communities towards these alien medical systems. The study also try to elucidate the reasons for the differential response of the Muthuvans and the Mannans towards modern medicine by considering the cultural, ecological and structural peculiarities of the two tribal communities. An attempt has also been made to understand how and why ethnomedicine and modern medicine still coexist among the Muthuvans and the Mannans.

2

Continuities in Traditional Culture

The data for the present study was collected from the Idukki district of Kerala state. The state of Kerala situated in the southern tip of the Indian subcontinent stands first in both population density and literacy rate. Kerala is a narrow strip of land which lies between 8°04' to 12°44' northern latitude and 74°54' to 77°12' eastern longitude. The state is isolated from the rest of India in many ways. The western side of the state is embraced by the Arabian sea, with a coastal line stretched throughout its length, while the eastern side is demarcated from the rest of the country by the mighty mountains of the Western Ghats. Kerala is divided into fourteen districts and Idukki is the biggest of them. Malayalam is the mother tongue of the people of Kerala, though in some places Tamil also is spoken.

Idukki district is divided into four taluks, namely Devikulam, Peermed, Thodupuzha and Udumbanshola. Except Thodupuzha, the other three taluks are situated in the mountainous region of the Western Ghats. As most part of this hilly regions are situated at an elevation ranging from 1500 to 6000 feet above mean sea level, this region is popularly known as the 'High Range'. The Western Ghats is a mountain tract stretching along the eastern part of India beginning from Maharashtra in the north and ending in Kanyakumari district of Tamilnadu, in the south. It is 1600 kilometres in length and decorated with thick evergreen forests and other dense vegetation. The forests give shelter to a large number of tribal communities, throughout its length. Its average altitude is 3900 feet above mean sea level and runs parallel to the western coast of India. 'Anamudi' which is the highest peak of the Western Ghats is situated in the Devikulam taluk of the district.

The main occupation of the people in this district is agriculture. The soil is very fertile and is ideal for the cultivation of tea, coffee, rubber, cardamom, pepper, lemongrass, ginger etc. This highland region gets abundant rainfall from both the south-west and the north-east monsoons. The average precipitation is about 1782 m.m. (1987) with wide variations according to topography and elevation. The 'High Range' which forms a part of the Western Ghats was fully covered with thick evergreen forests. But a large portion of this forest area was replaced by plantations of tea, coffee and rubber. Large-scale deforestation also occurred as a result of the construction of a number of dams; the hydroelectric project of Idukki is the major one among them.

Seven tribal communities are found in the Idukki district. They are the Hill Pulaya, the Mala Arayan, the Mannan, the Muthuvan, the Paliyan, the Ulladan and the Uraly. Among these tribal communities the Mala Arayan, the Ulladan and the Paliyan tribes are modernized in socio-economic terms, while the other groups are backward.

THE MUTHUVANS

For getting a clear and unambiguous picture of each tribe, it will be appropriate to examine the living conditions of the Muthuvans and the Mannans. As mentioned earlier the Muthuvans are found exclusively in the Devikulam taluk of the Idukki district. However, a few hamlets are found in the border areas of the adjoining Madura district also. A large number of Muthuvan hamlets are found in Neriamangalam, Adimaly, Munnar, Edamalakudy, Variyam, Mankulam, Marayoor, Kanthalloor, Bisonvalley and Surianelly. In a few places like Neriamangalam, Adimaly and, Surianelly they live in the fringe areas of forests. They have more contact with the nontribals in such places. But in places like Edamalakudy, Variyam, Marayoor, Kanthalloor and Mankulam they live inside thick forests and have very little contact with the outer world. The location of hamlets inside dense forests effects a geographical isolation from people of other cultures. The Muthuvans try to keep their traditional values and social structure intact in this sylvan isolation.

Visiting a Muthuvan hamlet either in Adimaly or Surianelly is not so difficult. To reach the 'Thalayarappan' hamlet of Adimaly one has to walk only for 30 minutes from the main road. The way to the hamlet is through a rubber plantation owned by the nontribals. The forest is seen only on one side of the hamlet while the other side is completely cleared for agricultural and housing purposes. 'Thalayarappan' is a small hamlet that consists of only 22 households. The houses are built closely in order to escape from the attack of wild elephants which may sometimes visit the hamlet from the nearby forest.

Usually an outsider is an unwanted guest in a Muthuvan hamlet. If the men are busy with some work, the visitor has to wait till they finish their work. The women never come out to inquire about the purpose of the visit. The Muthuvans are very suspicious about the true intentions of the nontribals because they were cheated by them very often. These bitter experiences taught them to view every stranger suspiciously. However, if they are convinced about the bona fide of a visitor, this simple and honest people will treat him with great affection and sincerity. They are a breed of naive, trustworthy and dependable people who never cheat anybody who seek their co-operation.

PHYSICAL FEATURES

The Muthuvans are considered as one of the best tribes found in this area in both physique and manners. Their bodies are hairless and they have only a thin beard and moustache. They are long headed with wavy hair and prominent nose and their complexion varies from very light to dark brown. "The Muthuvans are tall, strong and stout like the Sikhs and are most energetic and active. Their dress is distinctly different from that of the other Travancore tribes. They are courteous, disciplined and well mannered like the Todas of the Nilgiri hills" (Sengupta and Biswas, 1956 : 9).

Thurston found more than two types of facial features among the Muthuvans. He recorded : "I have alluded to the two different types of countenance; perhaps there is a third resulting from a mixture of the other two. The first is distinctly aquiline-nosed and thin-lipped, and to this type the men generally belong. The second is flat-nosed, wide-nostrilled and thick-lipped, and this fairly represents the women, who compare most unfavourably with the men in face" (1909 : 102).

Krishna Iyer puts the Muthuvans among the Proto Australoids along with other Travancore tribes like Malavetan and Kanikkar (1941:43). He considers the presence of blowgun among the Muthuvans as a contribution of the Proto Australoids (1941:46).

CLOTHING AND DECORATION

Among the Muthuvans, both men and women grow long hair. The men wear a turban on their head. The turban is a two meter long and half meter wide white cloth which is known as *'Urumal'* in their dialect. It is an identifying characteristic of the Muthuvans. Only men after their puberty are allowed to wear this head-dress. Now a days a number of men crop their hair and have discontinued wearing turbans. Their common dress is a *'languti'* and a loin-cloth. A white dhoti is the usual loin-cloth which is worn with a number of folds around the waist in the Tamilian style. Now a days they use shirts also. The youth prefer to, wear the loin-cloth in the simple style of the nontribals, in which the cloth is just put round the waist and tucked on the right side. The men also wear earrings made of silver or gold.

Women wear a brightly coloured long cloth which resembles the saree. The cloth after having brought round the waist and tucked in there, is carried over the body and two corners are knotted on the right shoulder. The whole body is covered by this long cloth. They never wore blouses in olden times. Due to the influence of modern culture, now they wear saree and blouse and only old women are following' the traditional dress pattern. The women wear earrings, nose ring, bangles, chains made of silver, gold, coloured beads or coins, etc. They decorate their hair with flowers and hair-pins of different size, shape and colour. The women always wear a comb made of a piece of bamboo or plastic on their hair. Luiz recorded that the designs on the bamboo comb consist of a series of hieroglyphics which are believed to be effective charm against diseases (1962 : 203).

HOUSING

All the houses in the Thalayarappan hamlet are one room huts. The house is built on a raised, rectangular mud floor. Wooden poles are used as pillars in the four corners. The wall is made of bamboo poles, rubble and mud. There is only one entrance in most of the houses; in some there is also another one at the back side. The roof is made of wooden poles and thatched with either wild grass or bamboo leaves. The room has an average measurement of 10' x 14' x 8'. There is a fireplace in one corner of the room, which is used as the kitchen. Sometimes there may be a separation for the kitchen. The floor is plastered with mud or cowdung. The people squat around the hearth and take food. In the night they put up a fire inside the room and sleep around it. They keep this fire in order to quell the biting cold in the high elevations. But the room will be filled with smoke which causes suffocation and irritation to the eyes. This will lead to the origin of lung diseases and can also impair the eyesight.

The Muthuvans used to put up a menstrual hut for women to live during their monthly periods. It is a small one roomed hut with an average measurement of 8' x 6' x 6' and is found at the back side of the main house. Women have to stay there for five days during their menstrual period. Other members of the hamlet observe pollution to them during this unclean period.

EDUCATION

A *'Balawady'* (nursery school) sponsored by the State Government is functioning in this hamlet. A lady teacher is working here. Children in the age-group of 4-7 are getting education there. They also get incentives like food, textbooks and a monthly stipend. Milk, egg and other nutritious food are supplied to lactating mothers and pregnant women, from the 'Balawady'. However, the children are very reluctant to attend the classes. As a number of children are present in the hamlet they prefer to idle away their time. The parents are also not concerned about the education of their children. Sometimes, they will employ the children to carry out some household chores.

A TRADITIONAL HAMLET

The living conditions of a hamlet situated inside the remote areas of dense forest is clearly different from that of a hamlet situated in the peripheral areas. The geographical isolation of hamlets inside the woods helps the people to preserve their traditional values, customs and beliefs. They are often more resistant to new innovations occurring in the society.

For experiencing the life of the Muthuvans in their original habitat, the investigator selected 'Edamalakudy' and lived there for three months in order to carry out the investigation. It is about 45 kms away from Munnar, a small hill station in the Devikulam taluk. There is an estate road upto 25 kms; then one has to walk about 20 kms through thick forest to reach Edamalakudy. It takes about 4 hours to cover this distance. The path is through dense evergreen forest inhabited by wild animals like elephants, tigers, bisons, wild boars, deers, bears, leopards, wild squirrels, monkeys and different kinds of birds and snakes. The presence of these wild animals is really a threat to life and a traveller for the first time will feel that he is in a quite unsafe environment. Even if one is not attacked by any of these wild animals and has completed his journey safely, no one can escape from the irritating, hostile assault of the blood sucking leeches, which, are plenty in this area.

The stillness present inside the forest is sometimes broken by the chirping of a bird or the echo of a waterfall. This curious stillness is much disturbing and one is not sure what danger is hiding on the way. A rogue elephant or a leopard can suddenly enter the way. So, one is very uncertain about the next step and often his life is at stake while undergoing such a journey. A stranger can easily lose his way and end up nowhere and if it is evening, his chances of reaching a hamlet before night are bleak.

Edamalakudy is not a single tribal hamlet as the name falsely indicates. It is a collection of more than 30 Muthuvan hamlets, of which Puthukudy, Periakudy, Shedkudy, Parappayar, Kanakudy, Kandathumkudy, Meenkuthy, Mulakuthara, Edalippara, Chembukulam and Aandavankudy are the prominent ones. These hamlets are embedded in dense evergreen forests covering thousands of acres. Each hamlet is about three to five kilometres away from the nearby hamlets. The investigator visited all the important hamlets taking sufficient risk of travelling through this elephant infested forest.

The Muthuvans of Edamalakudy who enjoy the sylvan isolation are less susceptible to changes than their counterparts living in the fringe areas of the forest. They try to preserve their traditional values even when strongly influenced by the modern culture through various government and non-government agencies. However, it will not be true if one says that the Muthuvans of interior areas like Edamalakudy are immune to changes and are preserving all their traditional values intact. Change is a universal phenomenon in each and every society and no group can evade from it completely. So, it will be fair to say that the Muthuvans living isolated in the interior areas are less affected by changes and are lagging behind in adopting various innovations than their counterparts in the outskirts of the forests. Resistance to change from the part of the Muthuvans is complementary with the non-availability of alternative opportunities to them from their benefactors. Anyway, an anthropologist can witness many of the old traditions at Edamalakudy which survived the tide of change by being isolated from the centres of civilization.

The traditional institutions like male and female dormitory, menstrual hut, temple, sacrifice of fowls and animals, observance of puberty and menstrual rites, use of traditional medical practices, reliance upon magical rituals to heal and prevent diseases, the office of the *Kani* (headman), animism etc., can be found in this region. The Muthuvans living here are proud that they still preserve these traditional values and institutions.

TRADITIONS OF ORIGIN

According to many anthropologists like Thurston (1909), Luiz (1962) and Krishna Iyer (1941), the Muthuvans are not original inhabitants of Kerala. They are immigrants from the nearby district of Madura in Tamilnadu state. When inquired by the present investigator the Muthuvans accepted this viewpoint and narrated many stories which supported this belief. Even though these traditional accounts differ in certain points, all of them support the view that the original dwelling place of the Muthuvans was Madura, and from there, they migrated to Kerala.

According to one version of the story, in olden days the Muthuvans were the citizens of the kingdom of Madura. They left Madura during the epic war between Kannaki and the king of Madura. Kannaki set fire to the Madura city to take revenge upon the king for killing her beloved husband, Kovilan. The whole city of Madura was destroyed and people fled to different places for their life. The Muthuvans ran away to the forests of Kerala. They also rescued their king Pandyan from the great calamity and took him along with them. They also took an idol of goddess Madura Meenakshi. They carried the idol of the goddess, their children and the household articles on their back. Since they carried the loads on their back (Muthuku) they were known as Muthuvans. *'Muthuku'* is the word denoting back in both Malayalam and Tamil.

After reaching Kerala, the Pandyan king departed from the Muthuvans. They started living in the forests of Western Ghats. Hunting and gathering forest produces were their major occupations in those days. Later on they accepted the 'Poonjar Thampuran' as their king. He allotted to them forest land to build houses and cultivate different crops. He ordinated a king for them who is known as *'Mel-Vakka'* and his abode is called *'Kiliparambu'*. The Poonjar Thampuran gave Mel-Vakka a sword, a brass pitcher and a bangle to wear on the forearm as his signs. According to Krishna Iyer (1941:25) the immigration of Muthuvans possibly took place at a time when the Telugu Naickans took possession of Bodinaickanur in the fourteenth century A.D.

THE MUTHUVANS' ATTITUDE TO THE MANNANS

According to the Muthuvans, the Mannans are an inferior group. They observe pollution towards these people. They will neither allow a Mannan to enter their house, nor visit the house of a Mannan. If any Mannan happened to enter a

Muthuvan's house, they will punish him and then desert that house, or burn it off. When a Mannan visits a Muthuvan hamlet he can meet the Muthuvans near the male dormitory. He can also enter the dormitory which functions as the guest house. However, the Muthuvans living near the border areas of forests are not observing pollution. They occasionally visit the Mannan hamlets, but seldom accept their food.

OCCUPATION

The traditional occupation of the Muthuvans is shifting cultivation or 'slash-and-burn' cultivation. This is the familiar method of raising crops among forest dwellers in many parts of the world. They chiefly subsist on ragi (Eleusine coracana) raised by this haphazard and unorganized slash-and-burn method. This method of cultivation is less productive and gives only meagre yield when compared to the more scientific methods adopted in the plains. But it has many advantages. It needs only very little labour and secondly it is most suitable for the ecology and is a non-spoiler of the natural richness of the virgin soil. They clear the forests during the months of February-March for preparing the field. In this process they cut down the small trees, bushes, bamboo groves and other undergrowth in a selected area and allow it to dry up sufficiently. Then they burn it and sow the seeds in the site after the first rainfall of the season. Sowing is often preceded by light hoeing with a long handled, narrow-bladed hoe. This hoeing will disturb only a thin layer of top soil and thus will not cause much soil erosion. Very often little attention is paid to the crop and there is no manuring. Often they return to the fields after sowing just to take the harvest. Some people come in the intervals for weeding.

After harvest the site is abandoned for several years, a new site being chosen every successive year until after a fixed lapse of time when the original site is once again thought fit for cultivation. Thomas (1963:367) recorded that seven years period is the customary lapse that the Muthuvans allow between two sowings in one site. The area will regenerate during this time interval.

The shifting of the agricultural field is accompanied by shifting of the residence each year. In recent times, this kind of free movement is checked by the strict enforcement of forest laws. As the area of the forest is depleted considerably due to large-scale deforestation both by government programmes and by the influx of people from the plains, the government has put many restrictions on the free movement of the Muthuvans. So, now a days they are forced to reuse the same site after a short interval of two or three years. This further reduces the yield due to the over use of the same site without manuring. This circumstance adversely affects the subsistence of the Muthuvans. When compared to the large scale deforestation by the government, the deforestation occurring due to shifting cultivation is much less. The deforestation by the government and nontribals is often for industrial purposes while the Muthuvans do it just for their subsistence.

Besides ragi, now the Muthuvans cultivate paddy, pepper, coffee, cardamom, lemongrass, sugarcane, ginger and tapioca. The Muthuvans are comparatively a lazy lot and avoids hardwork. In some places their land is under the custody of nontribals to whom they have given it on lease for a few years, after accepting a meagre amount of money. They spend a lot of time for fishing and roaming In the forest to collect various forest produces.

DIET

The Muthuvans' staple food is ragi. They grind the dried grains in a millstone and then cook the powder in hot water to make it a paste. They call it *'Katty'* and take it in the morning and at night. They drink only black tea at noon and do not take any other heavy food. They prepare some side dishes of either meat, vegetables, mushrooms or fish and eat it along with ragi. Now a days their eating habits are changing and they consume rice atleast once in a day. They purchase rice and vegetables from the market or from the food vendors visiting their hamlets. They also eat roots, tubers, fruits, mushrooms, honey etc. available in the forest. They hunt birds and small animals from the forest. However, eating the meat of buffalo, bison and cow is a taboo for them.

The Muthuvans always chew pan. The ingredients of the pan are the betel leaf, tobacco, lime and arecanut. They drink both black coffee and black tea and use sugar or jaggery to sweeten it. They grow ganja plant (Cannabis sativa) in the vicinity of their houses and smoke it freely. They say that ganja has so many medicinal properties. They drink arrack, toddy, brandy, rum, etc., and waste a lot of money for liquor.

SOCIO-ECONOMIC BACKWARDNESS

The soil of Edamalakudy area is very fertile and is ideal for the cultivation of cardamom and pepper. The Muthuvans own a lot of cardamom forests here. The cost of cultivation is very low. They carry out all the works by themselves and do not use any chemical fertilizers or insecticides. Even though they do not follow any scientific method of agriculture, still they earn a good harvest owing to the superior quality of the soil.

Even though the Muthuvans have a number of resources like vast areas of fertile land and adequate manpower to exploit the potential of this virgin soil through agriculture, they are still remaining as a very backward group because of several reasons.

1. They do not know how to handle money cleverly. They do not have any bank accounts and if they have any savings, they keep it in hollow bamboo bits.
2. They are illiterate or semi-literate and many of them do not even know to count the money they receive from the merchants.
3. The, unscrupulous middlemen and merchants easily exploit their ignorance and cheat them when weighing their agricultural produces.
4. In many places the practice of giving their land to the nontribals on lease adversely affects their prosperity. It is observed that in most of such cases the Muthuvans lose their land to the nontribals in the long run.
5. Their traditions and customs help to preserve the status quo and limit their ambitions. It

often supports a fatalistic attitude towards everything in the world.

6. Lots of money are spent for community feasts arranged in connection with marriage, death, puberty rites, festivals, etc., and for other expenses related to them. Even the more affluent people become debtors after such occasions.

7. They spend a lot of money on pilgrimage. A number of Muthuvans of Edamalakudy have visited the temples at Sabarimala, Palani, Madura, Thirupathy, Rameswaram etc.

8. They spend heavily on liquor and for modern articles like radio, tape recorder, etc.

These are some of the major factors contributing to the backwardness of the Muthuvans. But the Muthuvans are not aware of these handicaps which affect their progress.

SOCIAL ORGANIZATION

The Muthuvan Community is divided into six exogamous, matrilineal clans. They are known as the *'Melakuttom'*, *'Kanakuttom'*, *'Ellikuttom'*. *'Puthanikuttom'*. *'Thushanakuttom'* and *'Kaniyattukuttom'*. In addition to these six clans which are found everywhere, a clan known as *'Munnuttavakuttom'* is found in a few places like Plamala, Mankulam and Variyam. The division of the community into several clans is to regulate marriage ties. As the clans are exogamous one can marry a member of another clan only. The Melakuttom is considered as the most superior clan, from which their king *'Mel-Vakka'* is always selected. Each clan known as 'illom' is further divided into a number of sub-clans.

The members of each clan consider themselves as brothers and sisters and have a special attachment towards each other. If a clan member is in difficulty, then the fellow members will help him to overcome it. On occasions like marriage, death, etc., the clan members will help each other to carry out the functions successfully. When a clan member dies, all the members of that clan observe pollution for sixteen days.

The Muthuvans are matrilineal. The children of a man belong to their mother's clan. A man's property and debts are inherited by the nephew. The male children are named after their maternal grandfather, and female children after their maternal grandmother or aunt.

POWER STRUCTURE OF THE TRIBE

The Muthuvans have a king known as *'Mel-Vakka'* who is the formal head of the community. His official regalia are a sword, a brass pitcher, a bangle and three cubits of silk, and his royal residence is known as *'Kiliparambu'*. He always inherits this post from his maternal uncle. He is the guardian of law and order in the community and he looks after the welfare of all the members and protects them from the attack of outsiders. His assistant is known as 'Mutha-Vakka, There is also a hierarchy of other officials like *'Munnuttavan'*, *'Manthri'*, *'Valia Nedumpura, and 'Kudiyanavan.'*

Due to the influence of modern civilization and the abolition of royalty from the country, the Mel-Vakka lost his powers and is now only the nominal head of the Muthuvan community.

INTERNAL STRUCTURE OF A HAMLET

In each hamlet there is a headman known as *'Kani'* or *'Kanikkaran'* as its formal leader. He has the power to regulate the activities in a hamlet. He is the official representative of the people of a hamlet to deal with the outsiders. Usually a man inherits this office from his maternal uncle. But he must be an agreeable person for the members of the hamlet and also the consent of Mel-Vakka is needed before officiating him as a *'Kani'*.

'Thalaivar' is another official leader in a hamlet to assist the *Kani* in his official duties. There is another official known as *'Valia Elanthari'* who supervises the affairs of the youth in a hamlet. He has got a few assistants known as *'Chottupattakaranmar'* who help him in carrying out his duties. There will be a part-time priest in every hamlet and is known as *'Pujari'*. There will be also a number of shamans known as *'Vathy' or 'Manthrakkaran'*.

In each hamlet there is a council of elders known as *'Panchayat'* headed by the Kani of that hamlet. The male heads of all the households are members of the 'Panchayat'. It acts as a decision making body as well as the law-court of a hamlet.

STATUS OF WOMEN

The Muthuvan women, known as *'Muthu vathykal'* are very shy to face the strangers. If a Muthuvan woman happens to come across an outsider, she will quickly turn her face away and hide herself inside the forest. Thurston also noted this behaviour, "..... when suddenly met with, they (the women) make themselves scarce in the most surprising way, and find cover as instinctively as quail chick" (1909:101). Both young and old ladies are similar in their behaviour. The menfolk watch the behaviour of their women and so the women are much cautious about their dealings with the outsiders. The community is quite sensitive to issues relating to morality and chastity.

In the family circle, the women have a better position. They influence their husbands in cases of taking decisions. The husbands care them well. If a man do not show enough attention to his wife and children, others will not respect him and will consider him unworthy. When an outsider is present in the home, a good woman is not supposed to argue with her husband or the guest. The women are not members of the council of elders, known as 'Panchayat' and they have no say when taking any decision affecting the whole hamlet.

The Muthuvans are very reluctant to send their daughters to school. Even if somebody sends his daughter to school, he will not allow her to go after the age of puberty.

The Muthuvans used to get married very early; often before completing their teenage. As a result of early marriage the women get conceived in their tender age. This is detrimental to the health of both the mother and the child. It paves the way for large number of infant and female mortality. The Muthuvans are very reluctant to adopt family planning methods. As a result of frequent pregnancy and confinement the general health of the women is poor.

THE DORMITORY

The dormitory is an important institution in a Muthuvan hamlet. In each hamlet there will be separate dormitories known as *'Chavady'* or *'Sathram'* for unmarried boys and girls. In a female dormitory, the female children and unmarried young women will sleep at night, under the supervision of an old lady, often a widow.

Some of the old men will sleep in a male dormitory along with the boys and young men. A male dormitory is a big hall having an average measurement of 25 feet length and 15 feet width. Its construction is identical with that of their houses. There is a fireplace at the centre of the hall. There will be continuous fire throughout night and even in daytime during the winter season.

The Muthuvans use the dormitory as a guest house. The visitors will be accommodated in the male dormitory and food will be served to them there. One of the major functions of the dormitory is to prevent premarital sexual contacts between young men and women. Another advantage of dormitory system is that, after sending their children to dormitory, the married couples can enjoy a sex life in full freedom without any disturbance. Luiz observed "Muthuvans .... have '*Chavadies*' for youngmen which combines the features of a dormitory, club and guest room, so that they may have no contacts with the females and no knowledge of the sexual life within homes (1962:18).

Thus one can find that the Muthuvans are a group of simple, good natured people leading a semi-isolated life in the forests of the northern part of Idukki district. They have great respect towards their traditions and want to preserve these old customs and values. In their viewpoint the new values and innovations introduced by the modern civilization are not suitable for their living conditions and are against their ethos. However, the new environment created by the non-tribal immigrants from the plains, and the activities of various governmental agencies, are trying hard to influence the traditional beliefs and practices of the Muthuvans. The majority of Muthuvans who continue to live inside dense forests are successful in preserving their traditional pattern of living, even though with some modifications. The minority who live in the border areas of forests are comparatively more influenced by the new circumstances. The present study will analyse what is the overall effect of this tide of change upon their traditional medical beliefs and healing practices. The study will also focus on the interaction between modern medicine and ethnomedicine and to what extent it influences the health care of the Muthuvans.

THE MANNANS

The Mannans are found in the Devikulam, Udumbanshola and Peermed taluks of the Idukki district. Irumpupalam, Chattupara, Machiplavu, Adimaly, Korangatti, Mankulam, Variyam and Aanachal are the major dwelling places in the Devikulam taluk. Kattappana, Thovala, Vathykudy, Kozhimala, Murikkassary, Nedumkandam and Thoprankudy are the chief abodes in the Udumbanshola taluk. In Peermed taluk, they are found only in Kumaly.

In the Adimaly, Mankulam, Variyam and Irumpupalam areas they are found living in close proximity with the Muthuvans, Mala Arayans and Ulladans. In the Kozhimala area some Uraly hamlets are found near the Mannan hamlets. In all other areas they are living alone without much contact with other tribal groups. The Mannans are very sociable and mingle with others freely. They consider the Muthuvans and the Uralies as inferior groups, but they do not observe pollution towards them. They accept food from them and also intermarry with the Uralies.

Bensley writes about the Mannans as follows: "I enjoy many pleasant reminiscences of my intercourse with these people. Their cheery and sociable disposition, and enjoyment of camp life, make it quite a pleasure to be thrown into contact with them. Short, sturdy and hairless the Mannans have all the appearances of an 'aboriginal' race" (Thurston 1909:453).

The complexion of the Mannans varies from dark to light olive brown. They have dark eyes, wavy hair and both prominent and broad type of noses. Occurrence of two types of noses indicates a mixing of tribals with foreign intruders. Krishna Iyer suggests "where races with different nasal proportions are intermixed, the index marks the degree of crossing that has taken place" (1941:20). He found that the Mannan's nasal index comes only in the border of platyrhiny (ibid). Krinsha Iyer grouped the Mannans among the Proto-Australoids (1941:47). Their bodies are hairless and possess only a thin beard and moustache.

According to Luiz (1962:177) the word '*Mannan*' is a corrupt combination of the words

'Mannu' (earth) and *'Manushian'* (man) to conote that they are the sons of the soil, namely autochthons. However, a number of informants told the present investigator that the word *'Mannan'* denotes king. Actually this word comes from the term *'Mannavan'* which means king in Tamil. The Mannans claim that they were the kings of the forest in olden days.

THE MANNAN HAMLET

The Mannans live in hamlets known as '*Kudi*' in Malayalam. Each hamlet consists of twenty to hundred households. The houses are more widely scattered than those of the Muthuvans. In places where the government has allotted land, the Mannans have constructed their house in the centre of their property. A majority of Mannan hamlets are found in the fringe areas of forests, while some are situated in the interior areas. The people living in the centre and in the outskirts of the forest show very little differences in their life-style. Still, we can identify more traditional characteristics among the Mannans living in the dense forest. The geographical isolation is the main reason behind it.

The investigator visited hamlets which are situated close and far away from the centres of civilization. To get a close look on the life of Mannans the investigator first selected a hamlet called '*Chinnapparakudy*' in Adimaly which is about 4 kms away from the Adimaly town. A one hour walk through rubber plantations and a degenerating forest is enough to reach the Chinnapparakudy hamlet. On the way one has to climb over a steep hill to enter the hamlet. There are about 110 houses in the hamlet, scattered in more than 300 acres of land. The hamlet is encircled by mountains on all the sides. This is one of the biggest Mannan hamlets in the district.

HOUSING

The houses are built on a raised mud ground of rectangular shape. Each house is about 30 to 100 feet away from the next house. Most of the houses have an average measurement of 18'x 12'x 8' and there will be a separation inside the house. A small portion in one corner of the house is used as the kitchen and the big room is used for sleeping. Some houses have a narrow 'varanda' in the front side where guests can sit and talk with the family members. There are two entrances to the house, one in the front side and the other at the back.

The roof is supported by four wooden pillars and is made of wooden poles and thatched with bamboo leaves or wild grass. The wall is made of split bamboo and its leaves. The floor of the house is plastered with a mixture of cow dung and charcoal.

The Mannan house has no windows or ventilators and the room will be filled with suffocating smoke during cooking. Some Mannans put up a fire in the centre of the house during night, while many others are against this practice saying that it is not healthy.

The Mannans never sleep on a cot and always lie down on the floor. They believe that earth is the mother of all living creatures. So, it is a disrespect to Mother Earth if anybody uses a cot to lie down. She will be angry to those people who sleep on the cots.

The house and surroundings are always kept clean. A few hemp (Cannabis sativa) plants can be seen always in the close surroundings of the house. The Mannans used to smoke ganga (hemp) and also use it as a medicine. They strongly defend its cultivation saying that they are not doing it for any commercial purpose but only for personal use. The Mannans use utensils made of stainless steel, aluminium, china clay and clay in their houses.

In the Mannan hamlets there are no dormitories, the presence of which is a characteristic feature of Muthuvan settlements. All members of the family spend the night in their own house. If any non-tribal guest visits the hamlet, he will be accommodated in the *Kani*'s house which is often bigger than the other houses.

MENSTRUAL HUT

The Mannans observe pollution for ladies during their menstrual period. In those days they are supposed to live in a separate menstrual hut erected near the main house. This seclusion hut is known as *'Vannakkura'* in their dialect. During the mensus period the woman has to stay for 5 days in this separate house. She must take bath daily and keep her body and clothes clean. There will be a few utensils in the menstrual hut and she must cook her food using the rice and vegetables supplied from her house. She should not touch the utensils of the main house and must be contented with her separate utensils. During this unclean period she should not move around freely or talk to the males in the hamlet.

However, the practice of staying in a separate house during the menstrual period is gradually vanishing now. The investigator noticed that menstrual huts are absent in many Mannan hamlets which are situated in the fringe areas of forests. The women in such hamlets stay in a separate room in their own house. But they cannot enter in the kitchen during this unclean period. Food will be supplied to them in special plates and their movement also is restricted. Anyway no such change is noticed in the Mannan hamlets situated inside dense forests.

DRESS AND DECORATION

The traditional dressing pattern of the Mannans shows many similarities with that of the people of Tamilnadu. The investigator could not find any man who still follows the traditional style of dressing in which a loin cloth is tucked on the waist with a lot of foldings in the front side. When asked about the old pattern of dressing some men showed this style. Now the men simply wrap a loin cloth around the waist and tuck it on the right side of the body, which is similar to the style of the nontribals of the locality. They also wear cotton shirts and some of the youngsters wear pants and costly shirts made of synthetic fibre. The old men wear silver or brass earrings. They have no turban and the men usually crop their hair. Some shamans grow long hair which is their personal freedom.

Except a few old women, all other females gave up their traditional style of dressing. They wore no blouses in olden days and used a long cloth to cover their body. The cloth after having brought round the waist and tucked in there, one end is taken through the front side and passed over to the back through the left shoulder and the end of it is tucked either on the back or on the lateral side of the waist. As this cloth covers the breast also there was no need of blouses.

Now a days majority of women wear *'lungi'* (a coloured loin cloth) and blouse while staying in the house. When they go out of the hamlet they wear saree and blouse. They wear bangles, earrings, chains, necklaces and finger rings which are made of gold, silver or imitation of gold.

OCCUPATION

The traditional occupation of the Mannans was shifting cultivation. They followed the slash-and-burn method and would not stay in one place for more than one year. Now they have completely discontinued such mode of cultivation and are engaged in settled agriculture. Men and women are also going for wage labour in the nearby plantations. Their major items of cultivation are pepper, coffee, ginger, lemongrass, cardamom, paddy and ragi. Paddy and ragi are the traditional crops and they still cultivate them with nostalgic feelings.

When they have no work they go to the forest and collect firewood and other forest produces like honey, sealing wax, tamarind, arrowroot, wild pepper etc. and sell them in the market.

Sometimes they go for hunting also. But now a days nobody is seriously engaged in hunting and they do it just for fun.

Since Mannans are educationally very backward, very few of them get employment in government offices. Due to lack of education they could not enjoy the benefits of reservation of jobs. Anyway, the present generation is aware of the importance of education and a large number of both male and female children are attending the schools.

Now a days, the Mannans are interested in running small business establishments like panshop, teashop, etc., within the boundary of their hamlet. They get financial assistance from government for such ventures.

TRADITIONAL HAMLET

The contact with the centres of civilization is one of the decisive factors that intensify the pace of change among the tribal communities. So, after living in a Mannan hamlet situated very close to a small town, the investigator decided to spend some time in a settlement located in the dense forest. It was thought that the differences noticed in the two types of hamlets will be helpful to evaluate the influence of modern civilization upon the traditional medical practices of the Mannans.

The investigator selected a Mannan hamlet called '*Variyam*' which is located in the most interior area of a forest. It is about 30 kms. away from Mankulam, a small village in the Devikulam taluk. The '*Aanakulam*' river separates this village from the dense forest. To reach Variyam one has to walk about 20 kms through dense forests. This forest is inhabited with plenty of wild beasts like tigers, elephants, bears, bisons, wild hogs, porcupines etc. The path is the same through which elephants also roam in search of their food.

Besides Aanakulam river one has to cross two more rivers on the way to reach Variyam. There is no bridge over these rivers. In the rainy season these rivers will be flooded and no one can cross them during that period. In those days the Mannans will be completely isolated from the outer world. They depend upon tubers, roots and mushrooms to survive on such occasions. Sometimes they build temporary bridges, using huge trees and bamboo poles. But such bridges will be washed away within no time.

There are only 38 households at Variyam. All the houses are clustered together unlike in '*Chinnapparakudy*' where all the houses are constructed wide apart. The houses are built so closely in order to resist the attack of the wild animals. The houses are identical to the ones found in the border areas of forest.

The Mannans of Variyam are following some of the primitive ways due to the geographical isolation from the outer world. They are more superstitious and resort to magic to avert calamities. When anybody is sick they cannot take him to any hospital as the nearest hospital is about 40 kms away from them. So they treat him with herbal medicines and magic. They have no other option in this isolated area.

TRADITIONS OF ORIGIN

The Mannans have a rich stock of traditional stories regarding their origin. Even though one can notice some contradictions while going through the details of these stories, all of them agree in one thing, i.e. they are not indigenous to Kerala and are immigrants from Madura, a nearby district in Tamilnadu State. Their dialect, folktales, folk songs, dressing pattern, religious festivals, etc., support their claim. In all these things one can notice the influence of the culture of Tamilnadu.

Various anthropologists like Thurston (1909), Krishna Iyer (1941) and Luiz (1962) support the story of immigration from Madura. According to Thurston, "The Mannans are said to have been originally dependents of the King of Madura, whom they, like the Uralies and Muthuvans, accompanied to Neriamangalam. Later on they settled in a portion of the Cardamom Hills called Makara-Alum" (1909:452).

Krishna Iyer describes that the cause of their immigration is said to be their quest for food. "Being fond of animal food they thought that they could live comfortably on the Travancore Hills, which abounded in sambar, black monkey and other wild animals" (1941:25). When inquired by the present investigator, a number of Mannans supported this view propounded by Krishna Iyer.

In order to obtain reliable information about their origin, the investigator inquired with the Raja Mannan about it. Raja Mannan is the king of Mannans and the formal head of their community. According to him the Mannans have migrated from Madura in order to escape from the threat of war which was always present in Madura in those ancient periods. A large number of Mannans lost their life by participating in such battles. So, the rest of them migrated to Kerala in order to save their life and to live in a peaceful environment.

DIET

The staple food of the Mannans is rice. They take two meals a day, one in the morning and the other at night. They prepare side dishes of vegetables, meat, fish and mushrooms. There is no special food for the children. Occasionally they eat ragi and millets which they cultivate in their land. Generally they purchase rice from ration shops run by the government. However, a small percentage of people are still continuing the paddy cultivation. They drink both black coffee and black tea during the interval between two meals. They use sugar or jaggery to sweeten it. Occasionally they visit the forest and collect various tubers, roots, fruits, honey, mushrooms etc. They have complained that the availability of these forest produces is greatly decreased in recent years due to deforestation. Eating the meat of cow, buffalo and bison is a taboo for them.

SOCIAL ORGANIZATION

The Mannans are divided into two exogamous, matrilineal phratries. They are the *'Aravakudy'* and *'Panikudy'*. The clans of Orumakkadu Panikudy, Kandamalathu Panikudy, Malakkadu Panikudy, Adukad Nagamalayan, Muppankad Nagamalayan and Vazhar Nagamalayan come under the Panikudy. The clans of Thekkida Ailavan, Rajakattu Ailavan,

Chalukappattu Urukaran, Purampula Urukaran, Koompula Urukaran and Pulpura Urukaran belong to the Aravakudy. The mythological leader of the Aravakudy phratry is known as *'Varakkuraliyan'* and the head of Panikudy phratry is known as *'Kadadu Kumpilan'*.

These divisions are to regulate the marital ties in the community. All these clans are exogamous. The members of a clan in one phratry can only marry a woman from a clan of the other phratry. "The successive division of a community into two, four and eight exogamous groups seems to have been intended to prevent the marriage of relations of various degrees" (Krishna Iyer 1941:89).

Members of a clan show much unity among themselves. They consider it as their duty to help a clan member when he is in trouble. They help the household members of a dead clansman to carry out the burial and post-funeral ceremonies. They also observe pollution for seven days upon the death of a clan member.

A woman after marriage retains her clan membership and the children inherit the clan membership of their mother. A child is named after the members of the mother's clan. Descent is matrilineal. A man's property and debts are inherited by his sister's son. Due to interaction with the nontribals who follow patrilineal descent, the Mannans are also showing great affinity towards this system. Already people are giving their lands to their own children rather than to their nephews. Now, only the clan membership is inherited through mother without any change.

While describing the patterns of inheritance among the Mannans and other tribes of this area Krishna Iyer opined that matrilineal descent is now fighting a losing battle. Most of them are becoming patrilineal (1941:89).

POWER STRUCTURE OF THE TRIBE

The Mannan community had four kings, known as *'Malans'*, of whom only one is existing now. They are the *'Vadakkoru Malan'*, *'Thekkida Malan'*, *'Nattu Malan'*, and *'Varakku Malan'*. *'Vadakkoru Malan'* was the superior one among them. Each Malan had jurisdiction over separate territories. These separate provinces are known as *'Thalanadu'*, *'Adinadu'* and *'Thekkida Theruvu'*. *Only 'Varakku Malan'* is now surviving and is popularly known as the *'Raja Mannan'*.

The Raja Mannan is the king and formal head of the Mannan Community. The present Raja Mannan is living in the Kozhimala hamlet, near Kattappana in Udumbanshola taluk. His royal residence is known as *'Aayiraperumkuda'*. The regalia of Raja Mannan are a sword, a rope, a copper bangle and a 3 foot long cane stick, with silver rings at its tips. He inherits this office from his maternal uncle. He has the authority to conduct the trial of the accused and punish them if found guilty. *'Kuttiyathu Kolan'* and *'Kandameyku Edadan'* are the ministers of the Raja Mannan. They always accompany him wherever he goes out. The Raja Mannan also has twelve '*Kans*' (headmen) under him. The ministers and headmen execute the orders of the Raja Mannan. Each *Kani* rules over a particular hamlet on behalf of the Raja Mannan. The twelve *Kans* of the Raja Mannan are the following:

1. Koompilan Kani
2. Katta Thopran Kani
3. Purampula Kani
4. Edadan Kani
5. Aanakadan Kani
6. Kalkunthal Kani
7. Koran Vellayan Kani
8. Kuttiyathu Kolan Kani
9. Kularan Kani
10. Muthupuran Kani
11. Vekkiran Kani
12. Panikkan Kani

In the present age the powers of Raja Mannan are decreasing and now he is only a nominal head of the Mannan community. His power eroded after the inception of the democratic government in the country. Then the powers of the kings were replaced by the authority of the government.

INTERNAL STRUCTURE OF A HAMLET

A formal leader known as *'Kani'* is present in every hamlet. This headman has jurisdiction over that particular hamlet. His office is hereditary and the nephew will be his descendant. But the members of the hamlet also have a say in the selection of a *Kani.* After the death of a *Kani* or when he is seriously ill due to old age, another man will be selected by the council of elders as the new *Kani.* Their first preference will be the nephew of the retiring *Kani*. Only an able man, having ample knowledge in the traditional rules, customs, religion etc. of the community will be chosen for this office. He must be diplomatic and have the ability to mingle with the government officials and the nontribals. After the selection of a *Kani*, the Raja Mannan will be informed in order to get his approval.

A cane stick decorated with the red seeds of Abrus plant is the scepter of the *Kani*. His orders are executed by his assistants in the hamlet and he enjoys a number of privileges. He will be always invited to attend the important functions like marriage, puberty rites, post funeral ceremonies, etc.

Due to the increase of population a number of new hamlets have come up. In order to look after the affairs in each new hamlet, the members selected a new *Kani* for that hamlet. There is no limit in the number of new *Kanis* and sometimes the Raja Mannan may not recognize such a *Kani* as his official representative. They do not belong to the group of traditional *'twelve Kanis'*.

The power structure is quite developed and a hierarchy of officials could be seen in a Mannan hamlet. They include the *Aayiram Kudiyanavan', 'Varikudiyanavan', 'Periya-kudiyanavan', 'Ulanthari Kudiyanavan' 'Valia Ulanthari', 'Elayavattom', 'Thandakkaran', 'Thannipatha' and 'Keerapatha.* Each one of the officials in the hierarchy has certain duties and privileges. They regulate the activities in a hamlet. Some of them like 'Aayiram Kudiyanavan' and 'Valia Ulanthari' act as officials to enforce law and order among the people.

However, women are not represented in this power structure.

PANCHAYAT

In each hamlet there will be a council of elders known as *'Panchayat'* or *'Pothukuttom'*. The *Kani* will preside over its meetings and his residence will be the venue of such meetings. Women and children are not allowed to participate in the deliberations. All the common issues affecting the interest of the people will be taken up in this forum and solutions will be sought through discussions.

The relevance of the Panchayat is greatly eroding now. Due to the influence of modern culture people are becoming more individualistic. So, they sometimes refuse to obey the orders of the Panchayat and resort to their own ways to solve their problems.

SOCIO-ECONOMIC BACKWARDNESS

The foregoing description shows some of the prominent features of the culture of the Mannans. In socio-economic terms they are still one of the backward communities. One of their major handicaps is the non-availability of adequate area of land for agriculture. In some places like *Vathykudy* their land is either illegally encroached, or bought by the nontribals after paying meagre amounts of money. The Mannans are often cheated by the non-tribals in such transactions. In other places like Adimaly and Mankulam the Mannans have given their land on lease to the nontribals. Poverty, ignorance and the aversion to hardwork are some of the contributing factors which led to this situation.

Wage labour is the major occupation of a large number of people who does not have sufficient area of land for cultivation. They have to compete with the nontribal labourers for getting job in the plantations. It is observed that the Mannans are often the losers in this competition. Sometimes they may not get job for many days. Their condition is very pathetic in such occasions.

Very often the Mannans borrow money from the non-tribal merchants during the off-season. In the harvest period they have to give their agricultural produces to those merchants from whom they have borrowed money. It is observed that these merchants give only very low prices for the agricultural produces of the Mannans. They will also take a extra amount of money saying that it is the interest of the loan. The Mannans are not fully aware of this exploitation.

The Mannans have no instinct for saving money. Many of them usually get a good amount of money during the harvest season. On such occasions they will spend the surplus money by, drinking liquor, purchasing clothes and many other articles, or visiting their relatives in distant places. So, they will again become debtors in the coming season. The Mannans also spend a lot of money on occasions like, marriage, death, etc. On such occasions they have to arrange the community feasts and for this they have to borrow money or sell their land.

Generally the Mannans cooperate with the welfare programmes of the government. They are very eager to avail the benefits of such programmes. But, their poverty and ignorance often prevent them from enjoying the full potentials of these developmental activities. They do not have the patience or awareness to cooperate with long term projects. In some instances the selfish motives of the community leaders are a hindrance for reaching the benefits to the ordinary members.

Now a days a large number of Mannan children are attending the schools. But most of them discontinue their education after reaching 5th or 6th standard. Poverty and lack of motivation are the two major reasons for this large percentage of dropouts. In the Mannan community the male children will not get much parental care after they reach an age of twelve or fourteen years. Therefore, such children often go for wage labour or collection of firewood to earn money. Both the male and female children have to assist their parents in the household chores and after doing these odd jobs they will not get much time for study. As the houses are very small the children will not get a calm atmosphere which is essential for studies. In the night they cannot spend a long time for studies as the poor Mannans cannot afford to burn kerosene for such long periods. Generally, the Mannans do not like to send their children to the hostels for tribal students, which are run by the Tribal Development Department. The Tribal students get free food and accommodation in these hostels. Actually the parents want the assistance of their children in their daily life. In addition to this, they are not aware of the importance of educating their children.

In the present age many of the old traditions of the Mannans have been transformed and new values and norms have come up in their place. The traditional values, codes and customes of the community have lost their popularity and they are now existing only in the people's mind rather than in actual practice. The powers of all the traditional leaders like 'Raja Mannan', 'Kani', 'Aayiram Kudiyanavan' etc., are vanishing. A new breed of young leaders are emerging in their place who are literate and politically conscious.

Now each member of the hamlet has his own private property. He cultivates land and spends the money for his own private needs. They now imitate the materialistic ways of the non-tribals and the contact with them and various government officials have changed their mode of thinking and acting. Due to these outside influences each person is becoming more and more individualistic and gradually losing his affinity towards group life.

The subsystem of ethnomedicine is an integral part of the major system of society. So, when social change occur, the medical system is also bound to change from its own original self. As a part of modern culture, modern medicine also entered the universe of the Mannans. The present study will analyse the relevance of ethnomedicine, the role played by it in the healing practices of the Mannans and how this system is influenced by modern medicine.

The Table 2.1 shows the population composition of the Muthuvans and the Mannans and also the strength of a single household.

Table 2.1 : Population Composition Showing Age and Sex

	Muthuvan			*Mannan*		
Age	*Male*	*Female*	*Total*	*Male*	*Female*	*Total*
0-5	63	56	119	60	52	112
6-10	64	70	134	62	66	128
11-15	67	71	138	72	68	140
16-20	65	60	125	59	71	130
21-25	48	54	102	63	56	119
26-30	41	49	90	50	54	104
31-35	35	39	74	35	46	81
36-40	33	28	61	30	33	63
41-45	17	20	37	29	24	53
46-50	15	12	27	27	23	50
51-55	12	12	24	22	20	42
56-60	13	8	21	18	15	33
61-65	8	12	20	11	14	25
66-70	4	5	9	7	8	15
70 +	6	8	14	5	7	12
Total	491	504	995	550	557	1107

The Table No. 2.2 shows that a Muthuvan household contain lesser number of members than a Mannan household.

Table 2.2 : Strength of a Household

Tribe	*Number of Households*	*Total Population*	*Strength of One Household*
Muthuvan	200	995	4.97
Mannan	200	1107	5.53

THE MUTHUVANS AND THE MANNANS: DIFFERENTIATING CHARACTERISTICS

The Muthuvans and the Mannans possess many characteristics which differentiate these two tribal communities. Even though they dwell in more or less the same geographical region, their subsistence pattern is different. While the major occupation of the Muthuvans is shifting cultivation, the Mannans pursue with settled agriculture and agricultural labour.

The location of the Muthuvan and Mannan hamlets possesses many differences. Majority of the Muthuvan hamlets are situated inside dense forests. The people living in these hamlets have only limited contacts with the outer world. They enjoy the sylvan isolation and are very slow in receiving the innovations of the modern civilization. A small percentage of Muthuvan hamlets are found in the border areas of forests. However, they also keep a distance with the non-tribal people and try to preserve their tradition. This tendency for continuing their own tradition is due to some structural peculiarities of the community. On the other hand, most of the Mannan hamlets are situated in the fringe areas of forests. They enjoy little isolation from the non-tribal society. The Mannans by nature are very sociable and mingle with the non-tribals freely. The number of Mannan hamlets isolated from the mainstream are very few.

Presence of a strong leadership at the hamlet level is very helpful to the Muthuvans to continue many of their traditional customs and practices without any change. Most of the traditional leaders like *'Kani'* and *'Thalaivar'* are old people who want to maintain the status quo in the community. They have no appreciation towards the new innovations occurring in the mainstream. The strong leadership and also the authority of the council of elders (Panchayat) make each hamlet very cohesive. Therefore, individual freedom is very limited in the Muthuvan community and each member is answerable to its leaders. However, in the Mannan community, no such strong leadership is present in the hamlet level. At present authority of the traditional leaders like *'Kani'* and *'Aayiram Kudiyanavan'* has declined and they have become only nominal leaders of the community. This weakness of leadership encouraged more individualism in the Mannan community. Now the Mannans imitate the materialistic ways of the nontribals and do not give prime importance to the unity and cohesion of the community.

The level of acculturation is different in the Muthuvan and the Mannan communities. The Muthuvans, who still lead a semi-isolated life are less acculturated than the Mannans. The literacy rate of the Muthuvans is very low and they have limited enthusiasm to cooperate with the developmental activities of the government. They think that their present mode of living is best suitable for them and the innovations proposed in the welfare programmes will be detrimental to their interests. However, the Mannans are very enthusiastic to cooperate with the developmental programmes of the government and they get a number of benefits from them. Their literacy rate is much better, in comparison with the Muthuvans. A large number of children are now going to schools even though the percentage of dropouts also is high. The Table 2.3 shows the sex-wise literacy rate of the two tribes. The members belonging to the age group of (0-5) are not considered while determining the literacy rate. It can, be noticed that the Muthuvans are very backward than the Mannans in the literacy rate. Also the female literacy rate is very low in comparison with the male literacy rate.

The difference in the subsistence pattern has its own influence in the interaction between tribals and non-tribals. The Muthuvans who follow shifting cultivation inside dense forests have only little chance and necessity to mingle with the non-tribals. The Mannans who are settled agriculturalists in the fringe areas of forests and also wage labourers in the plantations have a lot of opportunities to interact with the nontribals. The Muthuvans who have limited contact with the non-tribals are less influenced by them while the Mannans who have close association with the nontribals are greatly influenced by them.

Many of the traditional institutions like dormitory, menstrual hut, observance of puberty and menstrual rites, etc., are still preserved in the Muthuvan community. But dormitory is absent

Table 2.3 : Sex Wise Literacy Rates

Tribe	*Illiterates*		*Know to read and write.*		*Std.V and above*	
	Male	*Female*	*Male*	*Female*	*Male*	*Female*
Muthuvan	340 (38.81)	411 (46.91)	78 (8.90)	37 (4.22)	10 (1.14)	Nil
Mannan	246 (24.72)	341 (34.27)	183 (18.39)	133 (13.36)	61 (6.13)	31 (3.11)

Figures in the parentheses denote percentage.

among the Mannans. The practice of living in a separate menstrual hut is gradually vanishing in the Mannan community. They are also not much particular in the observance of the puberty and menstrual ceremonies.

Definitely these differences between the two tribal communities may have their own influence on their medical beliefs and practices. A basic understanding of the social structure, occupation, level of acculturation and the general response towards the developmental programmes of the government will be helpful in analysing their medical practices and healing rituals.

3

Religion and Supernaturalism

Religion is a belief in the existence of supernatural forces which are beyond the control of man. Man seeks the help of supernatural powers, because, his everyday existence is surrounded by unpredictable and sometimes terrifying hazards. And there exists no adequate body of empirical knowledge which might enable man to cope with these hazards, by means of practical, scientifically proven or provable techniques. Religion fills the gaps in human knowledge and experience and so diminishes areas of doubt and uncertainty. Thus religious belief and practice may give confidence in the face of dangers which would otherwise be overwhelming. They provide institutionalized means of coping with such dangers, and even if these means are generally scientifically ineffective, they are satisfying morally and emotionally. According to Raymond Firth, "religion provides a referent for the explanation of many events in human life which seem obscure and demand a meaning.......... It constitutes a system parallel to and in many ways opposed to the logical-empirical systems of science (1971 :215).

Religion is a part of the life of the tribal communities and it must be analysed and understood in the backdrop of the hostile environment in which they lead their life. Their faith is both practical and strong. They have a lot of things at stake, as they live in high mountains in the unpredictable atmosphere of the wild forests. Also the resources and techniques they possess are quite inadequate to meet the contingencies of their life. This helpless situation tends them to bend before the supernatural powers from whom they can derive strength and assistance to tide over the difficult periods of their life.

The religion of tribals is functional. They worship their gods, not for the sake of mere worship. Through worship and by making offerings, they gain a rapport with their gods and get a number of things done for their well-being. Thus, they have developed a give-and-take approach towards the supernatural forces. They hold the belief that their gods are supposed to help them after receiving the offerings. They also believe that the supernatural forces will punish them through diseases, crop failures and other calamities if they fail to show due respect to them. Beattie, observes : "Very often ghosts and spirits are thought of as being dependent on men, as men are on them; there are rights and obligations on both sides. In such cases, the relationship, like so many social relationships, is thought of as involving reciprocity or exchange" (1964 :233).

The religion of the hill tribes of Travancore was a topic discussed by a number of anthropologists like, Thurston (1909), Gnanambal (1949), Krishna Iyer (1941), Thomas (1958) and Luiz, (1962). They found that the religion of the tribes was animism, totemism and crude polytheism. These tribals are found to be believers in the power of supernatural spirits and considered that their goodwill is necessary to lead a happy life. In other words, the supernatural spirits are regarded as potentially harmful unless they are propitiated. So, the aim of much invocation, prayer and sacrifice is to turn away evil rather than to solicit positive good, though both ends may be, and often are, combined. Krishna Iyer noted, "the religion of the primitive tribes of Travancore may be described as a system of animism or spiritism, and their attitude to the supernatural is one of reverential fear in the presence of certain mysterious supernatural powers and beings who must be propitiated or conciliated to avert ill-will." (1941 : 138)

Even though obscure, the tribals have their own notions of theology and ideas about the functioning of various gods. The religious beliefs and rituals inherited from generation to generation, form an important part of the tribal lore. The supernatural agencies are divided into gods, goddesses, village deities, ancestral spirits, hunting deities, agricultural spirits, household deities, malevolent spirits causing disease and danger and evil spirits like ghosts of people who met with an unnatural death. The concept of the shape and figure of the supernatural entities is fluid and vague. So the tribals never tried to make the statues or draw the portraits of their gods.

They had certain jungle groves in remote areas inside thick forests. They believed that these jungle groves are haunted by either a single spirit or a number of spirits. While passing near these jungle groves, they used to bow their head to show their respect. They will never enter inside these groves without a specific purpose. Usually, they will visit these groves only to make some offerings or sacrifices during the annual festival seasons.

The relationship between the tribals and their gods has two different and contradictory aspects. On the one hand they supplicate themselves to the power of gods and try to please them through propitiation. The gods are considered beyond the reach of ordinary mortals and the only way to get their favours is through complete surrender to their power. According to this viewpoint, man is a worthless creature whose destiny is in the hands of the most powerful god. On the other hand, man tries to control the power of his gods through special ritual techniques. In each tribal community there are certain specialists who are experts in the art of magic and they know the methods to control the supernatural forces. Each Shaman may have a deity or a few deities under his control and through their assistance he will be able to do a lot of things. He is functioning as a vehicle of gods and at the same time, is able to command them by ritual techniques.

As in all other spheres of tribal culture, their religion also is influenced by modern civilization. But religion underwent transformation in a slow pace and many of the changes are superficial in nature. Due to contact with the non-tribals, they got exposed to various religions like Hinduism,

Christianity and Islam. Each one of these religions tried to convert the tribals to their faith and a number of tribals became adherents to these religions. Among all these outside religions, Hinduism was much successful in inducting a large number of all tribals into its fold, while Christianity was successful only in converting a big section of *'Mala Arayas'* into its faith. In the case of Muthuvans and Mannans, the influence of Hinduism was very strong and it had reduced the relevance of traditional animism. Since Hinduism also was polytheistic, it was very easy for the two religions to mingle each other. They have accepted all the Hindu gods and goddesses and built temples for them in the Hindu fashion. They venerate the idols and portraits of these Hindu gods and goddesses inside their temples. They have also abandoned their old names and accepted Hindu names. As a result of the influence of Hinduism, they have reduced the practice of animal sacrifice and their priests are turning vegetarians during festival days. Some of the tribal priests are even wearing a sacred thread, like the Brahmin priests, while carrying out the temple rituals.

Even though Hinduism could overpower the traditional religious beliefs and practices, it could not completely replace them. The tribals still have faith in the power of their jungle gods, ancestral spirits and other household deities. They still seek their help when necessary. At present, one can see in each tribal community a symbiotic union of traditional animism and modern Hinduism, where Hinduism plays the dominant role.

THE MUTHUVANS

The Muthuvans are traditionally animists and they have a pantheon of jungle spirits, household deities, ancestral spirits, evil spirits, etc. They also worship the sun, the moon, the mountain peaks and some animals. Sun worship is a special feature of the religion of the Muthuvans. They have no temples and statues or portraits of their gods. They choose some upright stones, which are conical in shape with a broad base, and venerate them as their gods. They keep these stones on a raised platform made of huge stones, under a big tree. The stones, which represent various jungle gods, are sometimes painted with vermilion, ash or sap of herbs and flowers. Offerings are made when a difficulty arises and divine help is sought to overcome it. The usual offerings are flowers, fruits, little coins, twigs of herbs, agricultural produces etc. When confronted with a serious problem they may sacrifice an animal or a cock and sprinkle the blood of the victim over the stones.

In the present age, the traditional animistic beliefs are undergoing transformation and they give way to the doctrine of Hinduism. The contact with the non-tribals exposed the Muthuvans to the influence of different religions like Christianity, Islam and Hinduism. Out of these religions, only Hinduism could make a lasting impact on the Muthuvans. Due to the influence of Hinduism, now they have taken Hindu names and profess themselves to be Hindus. All the spheres of their religious life have been affected and transformed by Hinduism. According to A.A.D. Luiz "primitive animism and totemism have to a very great extent disappeared from among the Muthuvans" (1962 :206).

But it cannot be denied that, even though there has been a giant march of Hinduism into the Muthuvan community, still it could not completely replace animism and totemism. The Muthuvans of today follow Hindu teachings and rituals outwardly and yet preserve a deep faith in their own traditional gods and ancestral spirits. They accept all the gods in the pantheon of Hinduism, follow their mode of worship and celebrate their festivals. So a crude mixture of traditional animism and Hinduism is the order of the day.

THE CHIEF GODS

The Muthuvans worship two groups of gods. The first group comprises the traditional animistic gods whom they retain even after the influx of Hinduism. The various Hindu gods, they have adopted after their contact with the modern civilization make the second group.

TRADITIONAL GODS

The traditional gods of the Muthuvans can be broadly divided into jungle gods, clan gods, household deities, ancestral spirits, hunting spirits, deities of agriculture, evil spirits and gods causing diseases and other misfortunes. There is no concrete idea about the nature of these gods. No portraits or statues of them are available.

'Aadi Bhagavan' is the most important god, who will be propitiated first, while starting a worship or *'puja'*. *'Sukra Meenakshi'* is one of their household deities who is believed to be the incarnation of goddess *'Madura Meenakshi'*. *'Alangadan'*, *'Mankamada Thampuran'*, *'Madura Veeraswami'*, *'Kottamala Aandavar'* and

'Suriyabrahammamma' are jungle spirits, who always protect them while wandering through the forests. *'Ramar'*, and *'Pathakkulathukaran'* are gods they venerate to get success in their hunting expeditions. *'Uthampara Karuppannaswami' and 'Muniswaran'* are malevolent gods causing diseases, crop failures and other calamities. But their ill will can be averted through propitiating them properly.

Each clan has a special deity for looking after the welfare of the members of that particular clan. Each clan member will approach that deity first when any need arises, as he has strong faith in his assistance. *'Kotamala Andavar'* is the clan deity of *Melakuttom.'Nayamar Bhagavathy'* is the clan deity of *Kanakuttom. 'Thrikkal Devan'* is the clan god of *'Ellikuttom'* and *'Ramar'* is the clan deity of *'Puthanikuttom'*. *'Alangadan'* is the clan deity of *'Thushanakuttom'* and *'Pathakulathukaran'* is the clan god responsible for the welfare of the members of *'Kaniyattukuttom'*.

The jungle gods or *'Maladaivangal'* are divided into two categories. Some jungle gods are present in the whole universe wherever Muthuvans are living. *'Mankamada Daivam, 'Alangadan', 'Karuppanna Swami', 'Kottamala Aandavar', 'Thrikkal Devan', 'Ramar', 'Bhadrakali', 'Muniswaran'* etc. belong to this group. They have power over the whole universe and are venerated by the Muthuvans in all places.

The second category of jungle gods are present only in some localities, and they have power over only a restricted area. As their power is localized, they are recognized and venerated by the Muthuvans living only in that particular area.

'Nayamar Bhagavathy, Pathakkulathukaran, Oosimala Nadar, Aanakulam Bhagavathy, Chittattu Bhagavathy' etc. belong to the category of local gods. These local gods have some permanent residing places. Often they are found either on a mountain cliff or inside a jungle grove. The Muthuvans never wander around these places without any purpose. They consider these places as sacred and charged with the power of the deity. So any prowling into this private land of the deity is usually avoided and is considered as dangerous. Often they pay a visit to this jungle grove or mountain cliff during the annual festival season, to make an offering or sacrifice.

Generally all the jungle gods, except a few, are benevolent and they will help the people in their hour of need. But they may turn into malevolent ones if not propitiated properly. So they are worshipped periodically and special offerings will be made to them at the time of festivals. The male members of one clan will join together and then visit the jungle grove to make the worship and sacrifices to their clan god on the day of the annual *Pongal* festival in January.

EVIL SPIRITS

Evil spirits are a group of supernatural entities which are always malevolent. They do a lot of harm to the people even without any provocation. Young children and pregnant women are believed to be more vulnerable to their attack. They may bring diseases to little children and may drink the blood of a foetus leading to successive abortions. The Muthuvans believe that the spirits of people who meet with an unnatural death, like suicide or trampled by a wild elephant, or washed away by a flood or water fall etc. become evil spirits. They are known as *Chekuthan*, *Pey*, *Pishachy*, *Muni*, *Bhootham*, etc. Their attack can be averted through invoking the help of some powerful jungle gods which are benevolent towards people. Wearing of talisman charged with magical power, also will be helpful to prevent their attack.

HINDU GODS

With the introduction of Hinduism, a pantheon of Hindu gods entered into the religious universe of the Muthuvans. Some of them retain their identity, while others underwent transformation at the hands of the Muthuvans. They gave them new names and converted them into jungle gods. To cite a few examples, Lord Mahavishnu is called *Alangadan* or *Mangamada Daivam* and is considered as a jungle spirit, while *Bhadrakali* is named as *Vanakali* or *Adimakkari*. However the majority of the Hindu gods could preserve their identity. The chief gods worshipped by the Muthuvans are *Murugan*, *Vinayakan*, *Parvathi*, *Paramasivan*, *Sreekrishnan*, *Madura Meenakshi*, etc. Recently they have started worshipping gods like *Sabarimala Aiyappan* and *Guruvayoorappan*, who are very popular Hindu gods of Kerala.

TEMPLE

In olden days the Muthuvans had no temples to worship their gods. The abodes of their traditional gods were jungle groves, mountain cliffs and big trees. There was no clear idea about the form, shape and nature of god and other supernatural spirits. These supernatural entities were conceived as immaterial and, usually, as being diffused through space, or perhaps as not in space at all. But man always tried to associate these spirits with specific places in the material world.

Only after the contact with the non-tribal Hindus, the Muthuvans started making temples in their hamlets. Now in each hamlet, there will be a small temple, erected slightly away from the cluster of houses. It is usually made of wooden poles, bamboo and reed. The roof will be thatched with either wild grass or bamboo leaves. The usual dimension is 10' length, 4' width and 6' height. Inside the temple there will be a platform made of bamboo and is known as *thatty*. The portraits and small statues of Hindu gods like *Murugan*, *Parvati*, *Vinayakan*, *Sivan*, *Aiyappan*, etc., will be placed on this platform. Sometimes there may be a bronze oil lamp placed at one end of this platform. Small pieces of incense also can be found scattered over this platform. In one of the corners of the temple, three or four cane sticks, (Calamus rotang) can be found, with roots protruding from their ends. These cane sticks are the scepter of the priest and he will take them in his hand while performing some important *puja* or ritual. He has to keep it in his hand while possessed by a god or ancestral spirit.

WORSHIP

The Muthuvans are not very regular in worshipping their gods, for getting favours from them. Rather they go to the temple and worship them when confronted with any difficulty. So their worship is more directed towards averting the ill-will of gods, than invoking their blessings.

However, they used to propitiate their gods before starting an agricultural pursuit or during the time of a life crisis like birth, puberty or death.

In many of the hamlets the priest will make some *pujas* or rituals on every Friday morning. But only few people will attend the ceremony and nobody will give any importance to it. The priest will pray for the well being of the members of the hamlet during this ceremony. On the occasion of a worship a Muthuvan priest will first invoke and propitiate the three chief gods, known as *Aadi Bhagavan, Murugan and Vinayakan* before invoking any other god. Then the jungle spirits will be invoked. The newly adopted Hindu gods will be worshipped only after invoking these two categories. They have more attachment, respect and fear towards their own jungle gods than to the Hindu gods.

Usually in each hamlet there will be a priest to officiate the ceremonies conducted in the temple. The *Thalaivar* of the hamlet will be often the priest. His office is hereditary and he inherits this post from his maternal uncle. He is only a part-time religious specialist and functions as an ordinary member of the hamlet when he is not inside the temple.

During a festival season, the priest has to abstain from sexual intercourse and should not taste meat or liquor, to keep his body pure. Very often he will be possessed by the deities and other supernatural spirits during the festival days.

SWAMIKALLU

In the forests, where Muthuvans are living one can notice the presence of certain peculiar stones by the side of the jungle paths. These stones may have two to four feet height and are conical in shape with a broad base. They are placed upright on a raised platform, often under a huge tree. Usually only one stone is found at a spot, but sometimes two or three stones also may be found together. They represent Lord Murugan and some local jungle gods. They are called *swamikallu; swami* means god and *kallu* means stone in Tamil and Malayalam.

When a Muthuvan sees a *swamikallu* while going through a forest path, he will stop there and go near it, after keeping his sandals away. Then he will bow before it and pray to protect him while wandering through the dangerous forest. Then he may offer coins in front of it and no passer by will ever touch these coins, because of the fear of god. Or he may offer flowers or even the twigs of certain herbs. While moving through the forest, a twig found in front of a *swamikallu* is an indication that a Muthuvan has passed through that way earlier.

SUN WORSHIP

The Muthuvans consider the sun as one of their gods. They believe that by propitiating the sun, one can attain health, happiness and prosperity in life. So they daily offer worship to this benevolent god.

The Muthuvans used to get up before sunrise. Children will be woken up by the elders.

They believe that sleeping at the time of sunrise is a disrespectful act towards the sungod, which may invoke his wrath. The wrath of the sungod will be detrimental to the interest of the people. At the time of sunrise, the Muthuvans will bow before the sun with folded hands. They may sometimes utter prayers, seeking favours from the sungod. In the past, the Muthuvans used to start their daily agricultural pursuits or go to the forest for gathering forest produces, shortly after sunrise. But at present, after rising up, they sit around the fireplace drinking black tea and discussing various matters.

While taking bath in the forest rivers, the Muthuvans used to take water in their hands and lift it up towards their face. With the water in their hands they will look the sungod and pray to him for his blessings. Sometimes, they will take handful of water and throw it upwards, while propitiating the sungod. Those who know spells will chant them, to please the sungod at the time of propitiation. Like the sun, the moon also is considered as a god.

ANCESTOR WORSHIP

Ancestor worship is an important feature of the traditional animistic religion of the Muthuvans. The presence of ancestral spirits is a reality in the daily life of the Muthuvans. They believe that dead ancestors can influence the life of their living kins. After death, the dead ancestors are becoming powerful by attaining super natural powers, and their blessing can bring prosperity in the lives of people.

As mentioned earlier, after the death of a person, it is considered the duty of his sons and nephews to carry out the post-funeral ceremonies properly. In addition to the customary ceremonies which will be over by the 30th day after demise, the eldest son of that person must perform some rituals every year to remember the dead ancestor. Sometimes these annual ceremonies are conducted in order to please the spirits of all the dead ancestors. The blessings of the ancestral spirits will bring happiness and prosperity to the entire family of the dead person.

The eldest son of a dead person is supposed to offer cooked rice to ancestral spirits, once in a year. For conducting this ceremony, he must go alone to the interior forest with some utensils, water, rice and firewood. Then he has to select a good site, make fire and cook the rice. When the rice is ready, he has to clear some area in the ground and put a big leaf there. A plantain leaf will be used if it is available. After placing the leaf on the ground he will call all the dead ancestors of his family. He will chant a number of spells at that time, to please the ancestral spirits. When the ancestors are invoked, three flies will come and sit upon the leaf. The flies will be of different size and shape. One is called *Manneecha*, another is the *Kozhukeecha*, and the third one is known as *Varateecha*. These flies represent the spirits of the ancestors. So, when the flies are seen on the leaf, it will be presumed that the ancestral spirits are, happy and are ready to accept the offerings.

After the arrival of the flies, the cooked rice will be served on the leaf. The flies will fly away at this time. After putting the whole rice on the leaf, the man will return to his home. Nobody knows what will happen to this rice. No one is allowed to watch who will eat the rice and nobody can take it to his home.

Every year this ritual is conducted to please the ancestral spirits and to get their blessings. If somebody fails to conduct this ceremony, the ancestors will get angry with that man. The wrath of the ancestral spirits will bring diseases, crop failures, etc.

RELIGIOUS FESTIVALS

Celebration of various festivals to propitiate gods is an integral part of Hinduism. They are occasions for great enjoyment and they also give a chance to offer thanks to gods for favours received. Besides, they provide ample opportunity to escape from the monotony of daily routine. The Muthuvans follow the Tamil calendar, and they used to celebrate only the festivals of Tamilnadu. Their traditional festivals are *'Pongal'* in Makaram (January), *'Aadi'* in Karkidakam (July), and *'Karthika'* in Vruchikam (December). They do not give any importance to the Hindu festivals of Kerala.

Out of the various festivals celebrated by the Muthuvans, the *'Pongal'*, also known as *'Thai Pongal'*, needs special mention. This is their most important festival, which is celebrated for one week in the entire hamlets. It is the harvest festival of Tamilnadu and the Muthuvans also celebrate it during their harvest season. But they have modified this festival in many respects, to suit the peculiarities of their culture.

The temple of the hamlet will be thatched and repaired for the occasion, and various ceremonies, will be conducted there, under the leadership of the priest of the hamlet. On the second day of the festival, *'Pongal'* will be prepared by cooking rice in small earthen pots on temporary fire places put up in the temple premises. The people who had a vow, will make a *'Pongal'* and offer it to the deity. Those who had a vow to sacrifice fowls or goats will bring them to the temple and cut off their heads. The blood gushing out of the throat of the victim will be sprinkled over the *'Pongal'* rice and then offered to the deity.

In all the households, people will cook plenty of rice and meat, and all the neighbours and even the passers by are invited to share the meals. Members of each house are supposed to visit all the other houses of the hamlet and share some food, during the festival days. This will help to dissolve all the quarrels and hostilities that may exist among the members of the hamlet.

The feast, dance, songs and other celebrations show only one side of the *Pongal* festival. In addition to this, the festival has much ethnomedical importance. "The festivals conducted for the village gods are annual features or specially arranged either to ward off natural calamities, epidemics, or threat to the community by human agencies. (R. Nagaswami, 1980 :55)

During the festival days, the priest will be possessed by the deity and ancestral spirits, several times. Through the priest the gods will convey some orders to the people, which urge them to stop all the evil practices towards their neighbours and help them in their needs. They believe that if anybody violates this command, he will be punished by gods with diseases and other calamities. Thus the festival is an occasion to remind people to avert diseases, crop failures, and dangers by adhering to the right way of life.

Secondly, people could renovate their relationship with the deities through fulfilling the vows they have made when affected by diseases. This healthy relationship with the supernatural entities gives people a confidence that they will be protected from all diseases in future. Thirdly, the ancestral spirits also visit the people during festival days and are treated with new clothes, cooked rice, and liquor. Their goodwill can protect the people from diseases and other misfortunes, and ensure prosperity in life.

It can be noticed that, besides providing an opportunity for enjoyment and a change in the daily routine, the *Pongal* festival, also renovates the interrelationship of the members of the community and also their relationship with the deities and ancestral spirits. The healthy relationship with the supernatural forces, gives the people enough confidence that they will be protected from diseases and other dangers, in their future life.

PILGRIMAGE

Due to the impact of Hinduism, the Muthuvans are much aware of the specialities of various Hindu gods and their famous abodes. Visiting the holy shrines and temples is considered as a holy rite by the Hindus. After reaching the

Hindu fold, the Muthuvans also share this belief and imitate them in this respect.

The Muthuvans living in the fringe areas of forests are very fond of undertaking long journeys, often needed for a pilgrimage. The period shortly after the harvest season is regarded as the right time for undertaking such trips. At that time they have no urgent works in the field and also possess enough money to meet the expenses of the journey. The larger number of people are visiting the holy temples at Palani and Sabarimala. They also visit the temples at Madura, Rameswaram, Tirupati etc.

If their resources permit, all the members of a family will go together, otherwise the head of the household alone will undertake the trip, in the company of his friends.

The pilgrimages help them to learn a number of things. These are opportunities to mingle with people of different cultures and to see different life styles, places, vehicles, mode of worship, etc. The people who have undertaken such a long trip, are considered by their less fortunate brethren in the hamlet as heroes who know a lot of things about different places and about modern culture.

GODS AS REGULATORS OF GOOD BEHAVIOUR

The Muthuvans believe that the supernatural entities are watching each and every step they are taking and will reward them for good behaviour and punish them for bad behaviour. This concept makes them adhere to the right path of life. It is held that the behaviour of a man towards the supernatural and towards his brethren will be considered by gods.

The influence of the supernatural can be seen very clearly in their interaction with fellow members of the community. To cite an example, when a man finds honey, wild pepper, Boswellia gum or any other forest produce on a tree, he will either put a mark on the tree trunk with a sickle, or tie some thorny bushes over it. This mark will function as a sign for others, who may happen to pass that way. The man who finds a forest produce for the first time has ownership over it and nobody else has the right to take it from that tree. It will be considered by the community as a theft, if anybody dares to violate this custom. They believe that gods will punish that thief by sending diseases and other calamities to him. So, it can be noticed that the belief in the punishment of god, functions as a deterrent for men from committing an offence against his neighbours.

So, it can be noticed that religion is the basic and most important force working in the Muthuvan community. This institution is most resistant to the agents of change. Rather than a belief or dogma, the presence and active participation of supernatural forces is a living reality in the lives of the Muthuvans. Their concepts about the social mores, etiquettes, rules and regulations, crime and punishment, etc., are strongly influenced by their religious beliefs. As mentioned earlier, the peculiar condition of their habitat is the major reason behind this dependence on the supernatural spirits. With their own primitive technology, which is inefficient to offer them sure success against the adversities of nature, the Muthuvans found themselves in a helpless situation to survive in hostile ecological conditions. Epidemics, natural calamities, etc., threaten their existence and they know that they cannot resist these adverse conditions, with their own crude techniques. So, they invoke the assistance of the superhuman powers, which can help them to overcome the hostile situations. They salute the sungod while rising up in the morning and gods and ancestral spirits used to be mentioned several times in their conversations. While moving in the forest they bow before the *'Swamikallu'* on the wayside, seeking protection from the wild animals and other dangers.

The supernatural forces tend the people to adhere to the right path of life. Their propitiation leads to the celebration of colourful festivals, which redeem the people from the monotony of daily routines atleast for a few days. Gods also help them to tide over the uncertainties and anxieties developing at the time of the life crises like birth, puberty, death, etc. After their death also, they continue to exist in the community as ancestral spirits. Thus, religion is the all-encompassing entity present among the Muthuvans from their birth to death and also in all forms of social interrelationship.

THE MANNANS

As in the case of all the tribal communities of Travancore, the Mannans also are animists traditionally. They have a pantheon of jungle gods, household deities, ancestral spirits, hunting spirits, gods of agriculture, gods causing diseases and evil spirits. They have a well developed belief system and mode of worship to propitiate these gods. They had no well built temples for their traditional deities. The abode of these deities were, either the caves inside the forest, or a peculiarly shaped stone on the summit of a big rock, or a mountain cliff which was not easily accessible. A deity may have a fixed abode and it is usually worshipped only at that particular spot.

The Mannans have developed a reciprocal approach towards their gods. They often worship a god, and make offerings to it, while confronted with some difficulties which are beyond their control. While making an offering to a particular deity, people are expecting some favours from it. If they could not achieve the desired result from that god, they will discontinue the worship and seek the help of another god. Making offerings, or praying to the god, for the general well being of the individuals or community, is not so common. Very often the worship is directed towards attaining some specific needs.

The traditional animistic religion has been thoroughly influenced and transformed in the present age by the impact of other world religions like Hinduism, Christianity and Islam. Due to modernization and the immigration of a large number of non-tribals into their territory the Mannans are much exposed to the influences of these outside religions. Out of these different religions only Hinduism could make deep inroads into the Mannan religion and transform it thoroughly. Now the Mannans are Hinduized and their present religion is a mixture of traditional animism and Hinduism. But the more developed and well organized Hinduism plays the leading role in this symbiotic union. Luiz observed: "It does not appear that the Mannans were animists in the near past. They like to be known as Hindus and use Hindu names", (1962:179).

Even in this period of transition, it is noticeable that the traditional animism is still persisting in the Mannan community. But it has undergone so much transformation, that it now exists after many additions and deletions. Animism has borrowed so many features of Hinduism, and, has discarded some of its age-old practices. Hinduism also was modified in many respects after entering the religious universe of the Mannans. Hinduism practised by the Mannans has a number of differences from Brahaminical Hinduism. The success of Hinduism among the Mannans depends upon its capacity to adjust with the indigenous beliefs and aspirations. Thus instead of competition and rivalry, Hinduism and traditional animism are coexisting in the Mannan community with remarkable harmony. But, due to the dominance of Hinduism, with its colourful ceremonies, rituals, festivals, etc., the underlying animistic beliefs and practices are often obscure for a casual observer.

THE CHIEF GODS

The Mannans worship a large number of supernatural spirits of various denominations. They include their jungle gods, household deities, hunting spirits and ancestral spirits. After Hinduization they have adopted a new pantheon of Hindu gods. Even though they have accepted all the Hindu gods, to which they have been exposed, they possess a special reverence towards some particular deities. They venerate both the traditional animistic and new Hindu gods according to needs and circumstances. They enjoy more freedom and intimacy to deal with their tribal gods and call them immediately whenever any need arises.

TRADITIONAL GODS

The Mannans have a hierarchy of traditional gods. They always try to maintain a cordial relationship with these deities and invoke them according to the nature and urgency of their needs. *'Karuman Perumal'* is the supreme god of the Mannans. *'Thindiyi Kidakkum Thindilam Vellachy'* occupies the second position. She is a powerful, benevolent goddess, also known as *'Aanamala Devi'* as her abode is the mountain known as *'Aanamala'*. *'Vazhar Aandavan'*, *'Nayanachi'*, *'Uchanthool Vadakkan'* ,*'Sherkila Devi'*, *'Mala Devi'*, *'Shanthiyattamal'*, *Eruvakshyamal'*, *Meenakshiyammal'* etc. are some of the other traditional gods. Earth is considered as a goddess known as *'Bhoomi Devi'*. *'Pulla Vasy'* is the deity of agriculture and he is propitiated to obtain a good harvest.

There are a number of ancestral spirits, commonly known as *'Chavar'*. According to the Mannan theology, each individual will become an ancestral spirit soon after his death. *'Nedumpura Karanavor'* is the most important ancestral spirit, also known as *'Vakkalae Peatha Vakka Cheriyan'*. *'Sherkkila Karanavar'* is the second important ancestral spirit. *'Kattu Chavar'*, *'Kula Chavar'*, *'Muthuvan Chavar'*, *'Urali Chavar* etc. are some of the other ancestral spirits.

The Mannans also venerate snakes and the snake god is known as *'Sarppa Daivam'*. Unlike the Hindus, they have no jungle groves considered as the abode of snakes. Pictures of snakes can be seen drawn on the walls of their temples in some places.

Most of the traditional deities of the Mannans are residents of jungle groves and mountains. There will be a particular god for each locality and each god will have his own specific area of jurisdiction. Totally there are forty two jungle gods in the whole territory where the Mannans are living. Each god has an umbrella and a pole as his regalia. Each god has a servant known as *'Adiyan'* selected from the Mannan community. As a whole, there are forty two servants or *'Adiyans'* whose duty is to offer the due propitiation to these deities. Usually the head of a household will be selected as an *'Adiyan'*. It is his duty to maintain the goodwill of gods, by making the necessary offerings at the proper time intervals. Offerings will be made to the deities during the annual festival season. Then the members from all the households will bring their offerings to the temple of the hamlet and the *'Adiyan'* will offer them to the deity. Then he will invoke the deity and convey him the petitions of the people. Thus the *'Adiyan'* functions as a mediator between the deity and the people.

EVIL SPIRITS

Besides the benevolent gods, there are a number of evil spirits present in the pantheon of supernatural entities. They are malevolent by nature and bring a lot of hardships to the people in the form of diseases, crop, failures, abortion of pregnancy, attack of wild animals, floods, wild fire and many other calamities. Some of the benevolent gods also may turn into evil ones if they are not propitiated properly. The attack of malevolent spirits can be averted by offering them worship and sacrifices at certain time intervals. The assistance of ancestral spirits and other benevolent gods also can be sought when afflicted by the wrath of the malevolent ones. There are also some magical means through which an evil spirit can be controlled and its destructive power neutralized.

'Kalan', *'Karuman'*, *'Thuthan'*, *Thuttan'*, *'Yaman'*, *'Bhadrakali'* *'Muni'*, etc., are some of the evil spirits present in the Mannan mythology. *'Kalan'* and *'Karuman'* can bring crop failures and some natural calamities. *'Thuthan'* *'Thuttan'* and *'Yaman'* can cause diseases. *'Bhadrakali'* also known as *'Mariyamma'* or *'Valliyamma'* will bring diseases like small pox, chicken pox and measles. *'Muni'* is the most important evil spirit which can abort the pregnancy in a woman. This malevolent deity sucks the blood of a foetus from its mother's womb in the early stages of pregnancy. The body of the mother will be the abode of *'Muni'* in such cases. Magical cure is advised for this malady. Usually, the shaman will exorcize the *'Muni'* from the woman's body through some magical rituals. Then a fowl will be sacrificed and its blood will be offered to the *'Muni'* to quench its blood thirst. Offerings will be made in the temple to invoke the blessings of benevolent gods. They will protect the woman from a further attack of the *'Muni'*.

HINDU GODS

After the coming of Hinduism into the Mannan community, they have accepted all the Hindu gods to which they are exposed. Among these Hindu gods some are more popular and are worshipped with great reverence. The Mannans worship the Hindu gods like *'Sree Raman'*, *'Sivan'*, *'Parvathy'*, *'Ganapathy'*, *'Murugan'*, *'Mahavishnu'*, etc. Pictures of these gods can be seen in both temples and houses. 'Mahavishnu' is also known as *'Kadal Mulluran'* and is considered as the highest god. However, the most popular god is the *'Sabarimala Aiyappan'*. He is the chief deity in most of the Mannan temples. He is known by a number of names, like, *'Thekkum Pathinettampadiyan Aiyappan'*, *'Nadani Aiyappan'*, *'Cherkkila Aiyappan'* etc. He is also considered as a jungle god in some places. Even some parts of the forest are regarded as his abode. As a result of the free interaction between Hinduism and Mannan religion, some of the other Hindu gods have also been transformed into jungle gods, either completely or partially. The Mannans have more attachment towards these transformed gods than towards the ones who have retained their original identity.

THE GUARDIANS OF THE SKY

The Mannans hold the belief that the sky is four sided and has certain boundaries. On each side, one god is present to look after the welfare of the people living in the world. *'Patty Mycakombil Thinkallum Vellachy'* is the guardian goddess on the northern side. *'Kadal Mulluran'* is the god in charge of the western side. *'Madura Meenakshi'* is the goddess who guard the east. The southern side is looked after by the god, *'Sabarimala Aiyappan'*. There is no competition between them and all are concerned with the welfare of the people living in the world. According to the Mannan mythology, these gods have control over the sun and the moon and also regulate the winds, rainfall, thunder, lightning, etc. So they invoke these deities to get enough rain for their crops or when threatened by the natural phenomena like a tempest, flood or thunder and lightning. These are benevolent gods, always ready to help the people and rescue them from dangers.

ANCESTOR WORSHIP

Ancestor worship is an important feature of the traditional religion of the Mannans. They have strong emotional attachment towards the individuals who passed away from their group. Mention about the dead ancestors used to come in their conversations, frequently. They have an awe towards the heroic lives of their forefathers. The Mannans consider it as an offence to talk about a dead person contemptuously. The fellow members will regard a man as unworthy and sometimes rebuke him if he makes some absurd comments about a dead ancestor. They believe that a person after his death will become a god. He is called a *'Chavar'* which means, one who died. The ancestral spirit turned god is supposed to have superhuman powers and is regarded as a benevolent deity.

When parents reach their old age, they will usually tell their children, that even after death, they will be with them and protect them from every misfortune. At the time of burial, they will pray to the dead person to continue to protect the members of his family as he had done when he was alive. After the death of the parents, children will invoke them, and beg their assistance in guarding their crops from the attack of wild animals, and give them a good harvest. They will also seek the help of the ancestral spirits, when affected by diseases. They believe that the spirits of the ancestors, always function as guardians of their children and crops.

The Mannans believe that the spirits of the dead ancestors can become malevolent if their funeral and post-funeral ceremonies are not observed properly. The shaman has to chant the appropriate spells to appease the soul of the dead person at the time of burial. Then the relatives have to conduct the post-funeral ceremonies on the due dates. If they fail to perform this, the spirit of the dead person will become restless and return to his former abode. It will cause various hardships to the members of the household. In such cases a shaman can send this spirit back to his grave through adequate magical techniques and also by invoking the help of the benevolent gods. Afterwards, the household members of the dead person have to carry out the post-funeral ceremonies without any further delay to avoid any recurrence of the attack from the ancestral spirit.

TEMPLE AND WORSHIP

In the past, the Mannans had neither any idols or portraits of their gods nor any well built temples for offering worship. The abode of their traditional gods was, forest groves, rocky cliffs, mountain peaks, deep pools in the jungle rivers, huge trees, etc. They used to venerate these spots and make offerings in such places periodically. They also consider the animals like elephant and tiger, and reptiles like cobra, as divine and avoid killing them.

Due to the impact of Hinduism, the mode of worship of the Mannans has changed radically. At present, in each hamlet, they are erecting temples for worshipping the Hindu gods. The temple may be a semi-permanent building, usually situated near the entrance of the hamlet. It will be a little away from all the households and may be erected on a slightly elevated place. The average dimension of a temple will be about 12 feet length, 5 feet width and 7 feet height. The walls of the temple will be made of stones and clay, and are plastered with mud or lime. The roof will be thatched with wild grass or leaves of some reeds. There will be one entrance in the front side with a wooden door. Portraits and sometimes idols of various Hindu gods will be placed inside the temple on a raised platform about 4 feet high, made of bamboo and split reed. Bronze oil lamps, or sometimes electric bulbs in some advanced hamlets, are used to illuminate the interior of the temples. Incense will be burned and oil lamps will be lit while performing worship in the temple.

There will be one or two religious specialists in each hamlet. He may be a middle aged, ordinary member of the hamlet. He is known as *'Pujari'* which means a priest in Malayalam. He is only a part-time religious specialist and lives just like the other members of the community. He has to abstain from some food items like meat of porcupine and mountain squirrel, in order to preserve the purity of the body. During the days, when he has to officiate some ceremonies in the temple, he is not allowed to take food from a neighbour's house. He can take only vegetarian food, cooked in his house, on such occasions.

There will not be any *'Puja'* or worship in the temple, daily. Normally, the temple will be opened, for conducting ceremonies, only during the festival season. Some special ceremonies will be carried out in the temple if any major calamity like an epidemic afflict the people. Then special offerings will be made to the gods to protect the people from the epidemic and other dangers.

The priest will have to take bath before entering the temple. He will use white clothes and a sacred thread, just like the Brahmin priest, while performing the rituals. He will take away the sacred thread after completing the ceremonies in the temple. This is only an imitation of the Brahmin priests. The Mannan *'Pujaris'* have no specialized knowledge in Hindu theology, mythology and magic. They just imitate the Brahmin priests who officiate ceremonies in the Hindu temples. The *'Pujaris'* used to watch them closely, while visiting these temples for worship.

The Mannans pay occasional visits to the Hindu temples of their locality, either to participate in a festival or to fulfil a vow they have made to the god. They have deep faith in the power of the deities of certain temples. When afflicted by a disease or crop failure, they may take a vow that a certain offering may be made in a particular temple to overcome that difficulty.

After receiving the favour of the deity, they will fulfil the vow in due time.

In some households, the members have a particular spot inside their houses, for worshipping and praying to the gods. This place will be either in the centre or at one end of the main room. There an altar or *'Thatty'* will be made of bamboo poles and split reeds, and clothes will be spread over it. The portraits of various Hindu gods will be placed on it and usually a canopy will be made over it to prevent the dust from falling over the holy portraits. People used to pray before these pictures during the evening time or when any need arises. They will kindle an oil lamp before the altar at twilight and incense also is burned occasionally. Such praying spots or altars are found only in the houses of important people like, the *'Kani'*, the *'Vathy'*, the *'Pujari'* and the *'Aayiram Kudiyanavan'*. The ordinary members of the community have, no right to make such altars for venerating gods. If they want, they can keep one or two holy portraits in a quite unceremonious manner.

The Mannans take much freedom while praying to their gods. Usually, they pray to the gods and ancestral spirits very humbly and in a posture of supplication. But, if the gods did not heed their prayers, their tone will change and they will use abusive language in their prayers. Sometimes they will threaten the gods that they will discontinue all the worship and will not make any offerings in future if their demand is not satisfied.

TEMPLES OF TRADITIONAL GODS

The Mannans venerate a few places as the abode of their traditional jungle gods. Each jungle god is supposed to have his particular abode and his power is localized in that area. So the Mannans have erected temples for them, wherever they are residing. Actually there are no permanent buildings for these temples and only the Mannans revere these deities. The non-tribal Hindus pay no respect towards them. The deity is often represented by a stone with a peculiar shape, and may be kept on a raised platform made of stones, over a huge and plain rock or sometimes under a big tree.

Most of these temples were formerly located in dense forests inaccessible to anybody. Due to large-scale deforestation and immigration of non-tribals, many of these temples are now found very close to the centres of civilization. To cite an example, the temple at *'Pathinaramkandam'* is situated by the side of a public road and is close to a small town.

The names of some of the temples are given below. Each temple is dedicated to a particular deity.

	Place where the Temple is Situated.	*The Deity*
1.	Nerchappara	Pandyan Devi
2.	Pathinaramkandam	Kulachavar
3.	Mungappara	Nayanachy Muthy
4.	Ponmudi	Uchanthool Vadakkan

5. Vattukappara — Sherkila Devi, and Sherkila Karanavar.

Each temple is known by the name of the place where it is situated.

RELIGIOUS FESTIVALS

The Mannans show great enthusiasm in celebrating festivals. All their festivals are religious in origin and the important ones are celebrated during the harvest season. As people possess a lot of money during those periods, they can spend lavishly for the celebration. In the past there was no organized festivals among the Mannans, according to the traditional animism. In those periods, some celebrations used to be arranged during the harvest season or in connection with life crises, like birth, puberty, etc. All the members of the hamlet used to gather around to share the joy of such occasions. They will have a community feast along with dance, songs, etc., to celebrate the event. Gods will be invoked and their blessings will be sought

After Hinduization, the Mannans are much attracted by the well organized and periodical religious festivals of the Hindus. Till a few decades ago their major festivals were those which were indigenous to Tamilnadu. Due to the mingling with the non-tribals of Kerala, they now celebrate the popular festivals of Kerala, with great enthusiasm. The traditional festivals like *'Thaipongal'* are observed with little interest. Festivals of Kerala, like *'Onam'* in *'Chingam'* (September), *'Vishu'* in *'Medam'* (April), and *'Makaravilakku'* in *'Makaram'*, (January) are their major festivals now.

Out of these various festivals, the *'Makaravilakku'* celebrated in the Malayalam month of *'Makaram'* needs special mention. This festival is celebrated to extol the virtues of god *'Aiyappan'* of *'Sabarimala'*. He is the most popular Hindu god among the Mannans. His abode is *'Sabarimala'*, a mountain situated in the Pathanamthitta district of Kerala. The shrine of *'Aiyappan'* is found on the summit of a mountain, inside deep forests.

On the first day of the month of Makaram, a divine light will appear on the top of a mountain just opposite to the shrine, for a few minutes. The devotees consider it as an auspicious thing to watch this sight. The festival of *'Makaravilakku'* is celebrated on this day.

The Mannans also celebrate this festival on the same day, in their hamlets. In the night of that day, they will conduct a procession, carrying the portrait of god Aiyappan. A few men will play drums, while many others will crack fireworks, when the procession proceeds through the hamlet. Then special ceremonies will be conducted in the temple of the hamlet. The temple and surroundings will be renovated and decorated for the occasion. The people will fulfil their vows on that day and then pray to god *'Aiyappan'* and others to protect them, their children and their crops from all diseases and other misfortunes.

PILGRIMAGE

Pilgrimage is not an essential part of the religious life of the Mannans. But they are very fond of visiting various places and experiencing novel things, by carrying out trips. Pilgrimages offer them an excuse and opportunity to move out of the hamlet and see people and places. However, their financial constraints prevent them from initiating such enterprises, and only very few members of their community can afford this luxury. The financially sound members may sometimes visit the famous Hindu temples at Pazhani, Madura, Guruvayoor, Trivandrum, Rameswaram, etc. Large number of people every year undertake pilgrimage to *'Sabarimala'* temple to venerate god *'Aiyappan*. As this place is only about 150 kilometres away from their abode, many of them can afford this trip, at least once in their life.

MANNANS AND SUPERNATURALS

It is clear that, the supernatural spirits wield great influence in the life of the Mannans. Gods, goddesses, household deities, and ancestral spirits influence their way of life and view of life, and consequently regulate their behaviour, as individuals, and also as members of the community.

In their daily lives, the Mannans used to mention about the power of gods and ancestral spirits, and how they are protected and blessed by these benevolent deities. Always they are afraid to speak anything disrespectful about them. So, gods and ancestral spirits always play an active and decisive role in the daily routines of the Mannans. Before starting an agricultural pursuit, or a house construction they will invoke the gods and ancestral spirits, in order to get their assistance in carrying out that work successfully. When affected by a disease, or confronted with a crop failure, they will look towards gods to rescue them from that adverse situation.

The Mannans have no clear idea about life after death. They believe that the soul of a person will continue to exist even after death. The soul of a man who meets with natural death will become a god and this ancestral spirit is known as a *'Chavar'*. On the other hand the soul of a man who meets with an unnatural end like in suicide, or death in an accident, or getting killed by another man or wild animal, will turn into an evil spirit and its activities will be detrimental to the interests of the people.

It can be concluded that the religion of the Mannans is both functional and practical. Almost all their religious beliefs and practices have some strong relationship to the peculiarities of their habitat. Many of the rules and regulations imposed by religion enable them to adapt to the hostile ecological conditions, smoothly. The religious festivals help them to escape from the monotony of daily routines and also increase group cohesion. Thus religion helps the Mannans to lead a community life in peace and harmony by ensuring good behaviour towards their fellow members.

RELIGION OF THE MUTHUVANS AND THE MANNANS: SIMILARITIES AND DIFFERENCES

As both the Muthuvans and the Mannans are animists, their religious beliefs and practices bear some similarities. Their concept of the shape and figure of the supernatural entities is fluid and vague. So they never tried to make the idols or draw the portraits of their traditional gods. They also had no temples for their deities.

The living conditions of the Muthuvans and the Mannans have many similar features. The primitive technologies of both groups are not in a position to solve the problems confronting them, in their unfavourable habitat. This situation tends both groups to heavily depend upon the supernatural forces to thrive in this environment. Their religion is both functional and practical which help them to adapt with the adverse circumstances of their habitat.

Except these few basic resemblances, religion of the Muthuvans and the Mannans shows a number of dissimilar features. Each group possesses their own set of jungle gods, ancestral spirits, hunting deities, agricultural spirits and evil spirits. Their abodes and mode of functioning are different in many respects. The ritual techniques, the Muthuvans and the Mannans employ for the propitiation of these deities are also different. Sun worship is one of the characteristic features of the Muthuvan religion. But it is absent among the Mannans.

The influence of Hinduism on the traditional, animistic religion of the Muthuvans and the Mannans is very much different. Religion of the Muthuvans, living isolated in the dense forests is less influenced by the Hinduism. While religion of the Mannans, living in the fringe areas of forests, is greatly influenced and transformed by the Hinduism. Even though the Muthuvans accepted all the Hindu deities introduced to them and also use the Hindu names, most of their traditional religious beliefs, ceremonies and festivals are still retained by them. On the other hand the Mannans abandoned many of their traditional religious beliefs, rituals and festivals and adopted the Hindu values, ceremonies and festivals in their place.

The influence of the Hindu culture of Tamilnadu is less visible among the Mannans, when compared to the Muthuvans. While the most important festival of the Muthuvans is *'Thaipongal'* which is the harvest festival of Tamilnadu, the major festival of the Mannans is *'Makaravilakku'* which is a festival indigenous to Kerala. This shows that religion of the Mannans is more closely associated with the Hindu culture of Kerala than religion of the Muthuvans which still adhere to the traditional practices inherited from the Hindu culture of Tamilnadu. It is also noticed that majority of the Muthuvans undertake pilgrimage to various temples in Tamilnadu, like Pazhani and Madura. However, the Mannans show more enthusiasm to visit the temples of Kerala, like Sabarimala.

Due to the influence of Brahminical Hinduism, the Mannans have nearly abandoned the practice of animal sacrifice. On the other hand the Muthuvans sacrifice a number of goats and fowls during their annual *'Thaipongal'* festival. They also do animal sacrifice while performing certain magical rituals for healing a patient. Thus they have retained this feature of their traditional religion.

As mentioned in chapter three, the leadership of the Muthuvans is very strong who want to maintain the status quo. So, they will not allow the acceptance of noval ideas and practices in the field of 'religion also. On the other hand the Mannan leadership is weak and there is more freedom in the community. So it is easy for the new religious values and practices to enter into the Mannan religion.

The geographical isolation from the modern culture is another decisive factor influencing the religion of the Muthuvans and the Mannans. The Muthuvans, who are isolated in the dense forests retained most of their traditional religious beliefs and practices. They face more dangers and calamities from their habitat than the Mannans who live in the fringe areas of forests. The insecure atmosphere of the Muthuvans tends them to heavily depend upon the supernatural forces than the Mannans. On the other hand, the Mannans who live in a more safe and secure atmosphere find it less necessary to depend upon the supernaturals to solve all their problems in life. Due to the influence of modern culture they now employ rational methods also, in the place of or in addition to religious techniques, to achieve their goals.

4

Magic, Rituals and Medicine

From time immemorial diseases have been a part of human life and they sometimes have threatened the existence of human race on the face of the earth. Consequently, man has invented a host of devices through a trial and error method to control the vagaries of various diseases. The concepts of etiology of illness, methods of diagnosis and treatment and ideas of prophylaxis were developed and preserved as the traditional lore of every society. Most of this knowledge was acquired by men not intentionally; but through their experiences in everyday life they could evolve a body of practical, common sense knowledge. The basic character of this knowledge and the common feature expressed by the methods and techniques developed by them are that they are symbolic and expressive, rather than scientific and experimental.

The body of beliefs and concepts which existed in a society with regard to the nature, origin and treatment of diseases, was found always integrated with the other institutions and organizations of society. Religious beliefs, moral codes, social values etc. had influenced the beliefs and practices of etiology of illness and treatment, in primitive societies. Cultural patterns and religious beliefs, economy and morality, social values and medical beliefs are all found together to form the 'health-culture' of a community (Karna, 1976 :50).

It is common knowledge that, in many cultures, ideas and practices relating to illness are for the most part inseparable from the domain of religious beliefs and practices. The relationship with the gods and ancestral spirits plays a decisive role in the occurrence of diseases in a society. A harmonic relationship with the supernaturals often ensures protection from diseases and other calamities. So people make periodical offerings and worship to the deities and most of the annual ancestral propitiation ceremonies can be considered as ventures to ensure proper health of the community.

Medicine is a part of culture like religion, art, values, kinship, morals, economy etc. To understand the medical system of a group of people, one must study the culture within which it exists. To realize the effects of medicine on the sick, one must look at the ways in which such complex social and conceptual forces affect the human organism.

The various methods and techniques developed by the tribal people are not the results of scientific experiments. But most of them can stand the rigorous test of the scientific standards of modern medicine. It is understandable that expressive, ritual patterns of behaviour should be very much prevalent in simpler, technologically primitive cultures. Such simple communities have no scientifically proven method to tackle the adverse situations like famine, disease, epidemics and the ultimate calamity of death. So they are depending upon empirical knowledge and methods which are expressive and symbolic. Through performing the ritual procedures, people believe that they can bring about the cure of illness or ward off the attack of an evil spirit. For tackling such a problem, they lack effective action based on scientific knowledge. Beattie observes: "the people who carry out such institutionalized symbolic procedures or rites usually believe that by doing so they are either producing some desired state of affairs or preventing some undesired one" (1964 : 202).

The tribal people are leading their life in a hostile environment filled with a number of adversities. Evolving a formula to adjust themselves with the actual or potential dangers to their habitat is a question of their survival. A magical rite may provide a way of coping with situations of misfortune or danger with which there are no other means of dealing. Illness episodes are good examples where man finds himself in a difficult and insecure situation. In the face of actual or threatened disaster, to do something is psychologically satisfying and a way of relieving anxiety. When the available empirical knowledge is quite inadequate to meet the needs of the situation and where there is no scientific expertise to turn for help, men resort to magic for assistance, whose validity does not rest on experience.

Symbolism played the major role in the treatment of shamans. Their knowledge about the cause and treatment of diseases was empirical and expressive. As a result of the rituals performed during the healing sessions, the atmosphere itself became charged with mystery and suggestiveness. Most of the diseases were considered as having originated from supernatural causes and neither the shamans nor the patients viewed pharmaceuticals as any more important in therapy, than the rituals which accompanied treatment.

The ardent faith in the powers of shamans is a salient feature of the ethnomedical system. Nobody seriously considers their failures, and their successes are given wide publicity. Often the failure of treatment is attributed to the poor moral standard of the patient, or to the enormous power of the disease causing agent like a sorcerer or a malevolent spirit.

A man has to undergo rigorous training under a senior shaman, for attaining the secrets of shamanism like spells, divination techniques, healing rituals, etc. The community has some specific rules and regulations for both teaching and learning shamanism. There are elaborate initiation ceremonies when one begins to learn shamanism. Only people who possess good manners, character and honesty are eligible to learn magic which is considered as the most precious lore of the community.

Ethnomedicine of the tribals has essentially very little to do with medicine as everybody ordinarily understands this term, for the tribals do not share the understanding of disease processes as defined by modern medicine. For them medicine is a social institution enhancing every aspect of individual security-psychological, physical and social. People in the modern society view medicine as a branch of science engaged in the diagnosis, treatment and prevention of diseases. It has no interest in the morality, social status and religious life of a patient. It views disease as a natural phenomenon and suggests natural remedies for it.

In the past both the Muthuvans and the Mannans could preserve their ethnomedicine and other traditions intact as they were living inside the dense forests of the Western Ghats. Disease was present among them even in those days, as disease is but an expression of man's dynamic relationship with his environment. In those olden days they solely depended upon ethnomedicine to combat diseases. Hospitals and modern medicines were practically unknown to them. Religious beliefs were often intertwined with the medical beliefs and practices. They worshipped a number of jungle gods and ancestral spirits and they used to invoke them when their assistance was needed. The faith in god and in various magical rites was more important than the herbal medicine.

The traditional diet of the Muthuvans and the Mannans consisted of various food items available from the forest. Edible herbs, vegetables, fruits, tubers, honey, fish, crabs, tortoises, small games like deer, rabbit, squirrel, porcupine, wild goat etc., were the constituents of their diet. They also drank the pure water from the rivulets of the forest. They used to cultivate ragi, paddy and millets in the forest land. As they never used any pesticide or artificial manure the produces were very pure and unpolluted. All their food was obtained directly from nature. So it was pure and ideal for good health.

Since the people of those days consumed pure food and lived in natural environment, they were very healthy and the occurrence of diseases was very limited. They used to take many food substances without cooking. This habit helped them to save the nutritive value of the food. The cooked food items were usually taken immediately after their preparation and people never used to eat old and decayed food. If some cooked food was left in excess, they used to throw it away. These habits helped them to preserve good health.

There were no special midwives in the community and the old women used to attend the women at the time of confinement. Death of infants and also of women was common due to complications related to delivery.

In the past the variety of diseases was lesser than in the present age and they had remedies for almost all those diseases. The diseases were treated with the help of medicinemen and shamans present in the hamlet. They were experts in the art of shamanism and possessed a good working knowledge in the medicinal properties of various herbs and other plant and animal matter available in the forest. They had compiled this pharmacopoeia through a trial and error method and this knowledge was transferred from generation to generation by oral communication.

The Muthuvans and the Mannans use a large number of plant, animal and mineral matter for the preparation of various medicines. The plants and various plant derivatives form the major constituents in most of the medicinal preparations. As the abode of the Muthuvans and the Mannans is the evergreen forests of the

Western Ghats, they have close familiarity with the flora and fauna of these forests. The knowledge of the medicinal properties of different plants and animals enables them to select appropriate components to prepare medicines for the treatment of various diseases. It is observed that the two tribes employ certain common plant and animal matter for the preparation of some medicines. It may as a result of the similar trial and error experience with the available flora and fauna and also due to the fair chances of inter-tribal diffusion of knowledge on 'materia medica'. It is also found that a particular community may use a particular plant matter for the treatment of a specific illness, whereas the same matter may be used for another illness by the other community. Thus the same plant and animal matter are used for different illnesses and for variety of preparations.

Generally, the Muthuvans and the Mannans do not store the medicines. The medicinemen opined that the efficacy of medicine will be lost as a result of storage for long periods. So they prepare the medicines whenever they need it. They complained that it is very difficult to get all the components of some of the medicinal preparations. The deforestation resulted in the scarcity of various precious medicinal plants. The tribals always collect the medicinal plants from their natural habitat and they never cultivate them for their use.

THE MUTHUVANS

The Muthuvans have a well developed ethnomedical system. As in other tribal communities, their ethnomedicine is intermingled with other spheres of life, like religion, morality, social values, economy, subsistence pattern, etc. There are a number of experts in the community to carry out the various functions of ethnomedical system, like diagnosis, treatment, preparation of medicine, healing through magical rites, etc. They control the diseases through both natural and supernatural methods.

A 'MANTHRAKKARAN' - HIS STATUS AND ROLE

In each Muthuvan hamlet, besides the *Kani, Pujari* and other socio-religious specialists one can meet a *Manthrakkaran* who can be equated to the shaman found in the traditional anthropological literature. Through his spells, magical techniques and expertise about medicinal plants, he heals the patients, prevents diseases, wards off evil spirits, protects the standing crops from the attack of wild animals and sorcerers and thus functions as the guardian of the hamlet, who protects the people from all evil forces.

On most occasions, a *Manthrakkaran* functions as a shaman and also as a medicineman. Therefore, besides the knowledge in magic, he will be an expert in the peculiar qualities of medicinal plants. However, in some hamlets there may be another specialist medicineman known as *Vaidyan* who will be an expert herbalist. But he will not possess any knowledge in shamanism. He will restrict his activities to the collection of medicinal plants, preparation of medicines and the treatment of patients. He can diagnose and heal only the diseases arising from natural causes, while the shaman can diagnose and cure diseases arising from both natural and supernatural causes. So his status is superior to that of a mere herbalist.

A *Manthrakkaran* is an ordinary member of the community. He is only a part-time healer and he leads his life just as other members of the community. He commands respect from the fellow members of the hamlet for his knowledge in the art of magic and medicine. Any member of the hamlet can approach him at any time for receiving medical help from him. He is supposed to respond always to the needs of the people, even without considering his own inconveniences.

The status of a *Manthrakkaran* is below that of a *Kani* and he will not get any remuneration for his service. In a few places one person may function as both the *'Kani'* and the *Manthrakkaran*. But if somebody gives him some gifts to show his gratitude, he will not refuse them. So the medical profession will not fetch him a livelihood and he has to toil in the field like his fellow members.

VATHY

A senior *Manthrakkaran* is known as a *Vathy*. Through many years of experience he will be a great expert in shamanism. Usually *Vathykal* (pl) are old people who command much respect among the members of the hamlet. The ordinary members of the hamlet have a feeling of fear and awe towards them. The number of *Vathykal* is limited when compared to that of *Manthrakkaranmar* (pl). There may not be a *Vathy* in each and every hamlet though there may be more than one *Manthrakkaranmar*.

Usually each *Vathy* will have a number of disciples. They may be either his nephews, close relatives or sometimes his own sons. They are his apprentices, who hang around him to learn the art of shamanism which is known as *Vicha* in their dialect. The word *Vicha* must have evolved from the Malayalam word *Vidya* which denotes knowledge, technique, etc. The Muthuvans consider magic as the most precious knowledge and those who are experts in this art are considered as great people.

The *Vathykal* are divided into four categories, according to the nature of the problems they deal with. Each one has a specialized area of knowledge and an exclusive responsibility in his particular field. *Puli Vathy*, *Aana Vathy*, *Anther Vathy* and *Aakaya Vathy* are four types of *Vathykal* found in the Muthuvan community. *Aana Vathy* controls the elephants by his spells and thus protects the people from the attack of wild elephants. *Puli Vathy* saves the people from the attack of leopards and tigers. *Anther Vathy* is an expert in those spells and techniques by which he can control malevolent spirits and heal all the diseases caused by them. *Aakaya Vathy* can control deities and ancestral spirits through his spells and magical rites and can protect the people from epidemics like measles, chickenpox, cholera etc. He gets the power to control smallpox from the goddess *Mariyamma*.

Each clan will have a special household deity known as *Kula Devatha*. This deity will be the household deity of the *Vathy* also. The *Vathy* will also invoke the ancestral spirits of his clan when need arises. So, the power of the *Vathy* comes from the clan deity and the ancestral spirits.

Thus a Vathy is only an ordinary mortal and he carries out the magical cures and other superhuman miracles by the power of the supernatural forces. If a magical rite is to be successful, first he will have to invoke the blessings of benevolent gods like *Aadi Bhagavan, Shri Krishnan* and *Arjunan*. Then he will invoke the clan deity, local jungle gods, ancestral spirits and the seven *Kannikal*. When invoked by chanting spells, these supernatural beings will come and soon the *Vathy* will be possessed by them. Afterwards, the *Vathy* will be functioning by the power of these supernatural entities. Thus the *Vathy* is acting only as a medium through which the power of supernaturals comes and functions among the people.

TEACHING MAGIC

Generally, a *Vathy* teaches his magical techniques to his nephew rather than to his own son. The nephew belongs to the same clan of the *Vathy*, while the son belongs to his wife's clan. By teaching magic to a nephew, the magical techniques of that clan can be retained with it. Some of the important magical secrets are generally preserved and shared among the members of one clan. The clan members are proud of this heritage.

If a nephew is not available with talents to acquire the magical skills, an able son will be chosen as a candidate to learn magic. Now a days no *Vathy* follows a strict rule of inheritance for teaching magic. So even a candidate who has no blood relationship with the *Vathy* can be taught magic if he is found able to learn. Very often there may be more than one candidate for studying magic at a time.

Teaching will be started when the candidate attains an age of around forty years and if he possesses a good character. The teacher will watch his future student for a certain period of time, to know whether he possesses the ability to learn the secrets of magic and utilize it for the welfare of the community. After teaching the preliminary lessons of magic the teacher will again watch the dealings of the student with other members and especially to the needy people of the community. It will be noted whether he is willing to help the people who are afflicted by diseases and other misfortunes. If the behaviour of the student is found satisfactory, then all the important techniques of magic will be taught to him.

There are some customary functions on the first day of learning. On that day both the teacher and his students will rise in the early morning and go to a nearby river. They are not allowed to take any food that morning. On reaching the river, the teacher will stand in the water, chanting spells and looking upwards with half-closed eyes. Then the students will gather around the teacher and salute him. Afterwards, they have to immerse themselves three times in the water. Each time they have to drink one mouthful of water. They consider this water as the holy milk of goddess *Parvathy*. After taking bath, the teacher and the students will return to the hamlet.

The students have to take an oath before starting the learning process. They have to stand in water, neck-deep while taking the oath. The oath is like this, "We will be ready to visit a patient's residence and help him whenever called by his people, at whatever time, even in the midnight. We will not refuse to offer treatment to anybody, even to a man who has molested our wives, or killed our children. We pledge that we will always adhere to truth, justice and charity till our last breath." The learners have to keep this oath in their whole life and live according to its spirit. If somebody violates the conditions of the oath, god and ancestral spirits will punish him and consequently, the efficacy of his magic will be lost.

After reaching the hamlet, the students will clear some area outside the hamlet and erect an elevated, square shaped ground, surrounded with stones. This stage is known as '*Kalava*'. The students will then visit the teacher and offer him some gifts or *Dakshina* as a token of their respect and gratitude. The *Dakshina* will consist of three betel leaves, a ripe arecanut, a tobacco leaf and a one rupee coin. Such offerings will be made to the teachers of the *Vathy* also. Offerings will be made in the temple of the hamlet for pleasing the jungle gods and ancestral spirits.

Then the teacher along with the students will go to the *Kalava*. Those who want to learn magic have to stand on the *Kalava*. The teacher will sing a song loudly, describing some of the basic principles of their magic. In that song, he will also praise god Shiva, goddess Parvathy and the Earth goddess. The initial stages of learning magic will be carried out publicly. Other people of the hamlet can watch the proceedings of this big event by standing a little apart. Only the people who stand on the *kalava* have the right to learn what the teacher is saying. But the later stages of magic are not taught publicly. Usually the teacher along with his students will go to the interior forests, occasionally. There he will teach them the secrets of magic without being overheard by anybody.

The *Vathy* has got a number of supernatural aids, besides the gods and ancestral spirits. In the Muthuvan cosmology, there are certain supernatural beings known as *Kannikal* ('Kanni', singular). They have no definite form and are supposed to be very beautiful, white complexioned females. They resemble the angels of Christian mythology. They can take the shape of birds, butterflies, wind, etc. There are seven *Kannikal* according to the Muthuvan cosmology. Their status is inferior to gods, but always superior to mortals.

The *Vathy* can invoke the *Kannikal* through chanting certain spells. He carries out many of the magical rites with their assistance. When a student stands on the *Kalva*, the *Vathy* will invoke the *Kannikal* through a spell and one of them will possess the student. After being possessed by the *Kanni* the student will be able to grasp easily what his teacher tells him. The ancestral spirits, especially the spirits of the dead *Vathykal* of that clan, will be invoked on the first day of teaching magic. This is to seek their blessings for the new students. The spirits of these dead *Vathykal* will help a *Vathy* to teach his students efficiently.

TRANSFER OF MAGIC

Usually a *Vathy* will reveal the most important spells and magical techniques only when he is very old and approaching his death. Till that time he will keep the secrets to himself.

Very often a *Vathy* will die without transferring all the important magical formulae to another man. However, in his last days, he will tell his fellow members, that he wants to bequeath all his magical knowledge to a particular disciple of his. Only that man has the right to receive the important magical spells and techniques from his teacher.

There are certain techniques, by which a man can attain the magical powers even from a dead *Vathy*. In such cases, soon after washing, corpse will be laid on a mat on the floor. Afterwards, the man who has the right to inherit the deadman's magical powers will come forward and bow before the corpse. He will then chant some spells to please the spirits of dead ancestors and of the dead *Vathy*. Then he will rub the corpse from head to leg, three times, with his hands. By this method all the magical powers of the *Vathy* will come to be accumulated on the great toes of his feet. Then he will suck the great toes of the corpse simultaneously. It is believed that while sucking the great toes, all the magical powers of the dead *Vathy* will leave the corpse and enter the body of his disciple. The power is taken from the corpse, just before its burial.

FENCE OF 'MANTHRAKKARAN'

Ramar, Karuppannaswami and *Bhadrakali* are the important jungle gods invoked by a *Manthrakkaran* to protect the people from diseases. With the help of these benevolent gods, the *Manthrakkaran* will catch the evil spirits and destroy their power. His magical rituals are charged with expressive symbolism and are very suggestive in nature. So they can have a psychological impact on the patient and on his relatives. After the warding off ceremony, a patient will soon recover from his illness.

In order to prevent the attack of the evil spirits and sorcerers in future, the *Manthrakkaran* will erect fences around the hamlet. These fences are supposed to be made of steel and fire, and are invisible to the eyes of ordinary mortals. Whosoever touches this fence is assumed to die immediately. This fence is a protective device against the attack of both evil spirits and sorcerers. After the erection of this fence, no evil forces can enter the hamlet and attack the people with diseases, crop failures and other calamities. So this protective fence can be rightly called a prophylactic measure to save the people from diseases.

COMMON CONCEPTS OF ETIOLOGY

The Muthuvans have a number of concepts regarding the etiology of illness. This includes both natural and supernatural causes of disease. From the nature of one disease they will diagnose the etiology of the malady. However, beliefs in the supernatural causes of illness are more prevalent among the Muthuvans than among the Mannans. Sometimes, the Muthuvans even ignore the natural causes behind the occurrence of a disease and believe that they are also signs of the attack of some supernatural forces. Some categories of illness are assumed to be the exclusive result of supernatural attack while some others are the result of only natural causes.

NATURAL CAUSES

According to the Muthuvans change in the nature and quality of diet is the main reason for the occurrence of diseases. In the past the Muthuvans were eating only the food available from the forest. While going on a journey, they used to take cooked food with them and considered the food available in the hotels as polluted. The food available in the forest was pure and unpolluted and very suitable for health. But now they have given up the old diet and depend upon the food items available in the market. They also consume the rice available from the ration shops of the state government. Due to large-scale deforestation, the availability of food from the forests has been greatly reduced. They say that their health has suffered due to the intake of this adulterated and polluted food. Due to the deterioration of health their body is now more vulnerable to diseases.

Excessive exposure to hot sun, rain and cold is another natural cause for the occurrence of diseases. The rigorous climatic conditions adversely affect the health of the body and the person becomes weak and vulnerable to the attack of diseases. Old age and overwork are also considered as reasons for the affliction of diseases.

SUPERNATURAL CAUSES

The supernatural causes of diseases are more when compared to the natural causes. Wrath of deities and ancestral spirits is one of the main causes of illness. Possession of evil spirits, soul-loss, violation of taboos and sorcery are some of the other major causes for the occurrence of diseases.

(a) Anger of God and Disease

The Muthuvans believe that, for maintaining the general well-being and prosperity of the members of a hamlet, they have to keep a good, harmonious relationship with the gods and ancestral spirits. The gods will give a lot of favours to the people if they are propitiated properly. But the lack of worship will incur the wrath of the gods and even benevolent gods will turn into malevolent ones. The anger of a god is the usual reason for the origin of diseases. The gods will get angry when the people provoke them by doing something against their interest, or when they harm their neighbours with or without a reason.

(b) Ancestral spirits and disease

If the post-funeral ceremonies of a person are not conducted properly and in due time, one of his children will get sick, thirty days after his parent's death. Usually he will suffer from acute fever and headache which could not be controlled by the herbal medicines. A *Manthrakkaran* can find out the cause and can cure the disease through proper magical techniques.

Performance of the post-funeral ceremonies is the only remedy for the permanent cure of the disease. In addition to this, special offerings of liquor, cloth and cooked rice also must be made to please the ancestral spirit. Then they will pray to the dead ancestors to forgive their lapse and stop punishing them. After receiving the offerings the dead ancestors will be satisfied and then they will leave the body of the patient. Soon he will recover from his illness.

In order to keep the ancestors pleased, periodical offerings will be made. Usually such offerings are made at the time of annual festivals. Keeping a good relationship with the dead ancestors will ensure to the Muthuvans, protection from diseases and other calamities.

(c) Evil spirits and disease

There are a number of evil spirits like, *Chekuthan, Pey, Pishachy, Muni,* etc., in the Muthuvan religion. All of them are malevolent and cause various hardships like illness, accidents, crop failures, etc. to the people. The Muthuvans believe that some of the isolated corners in the dense forest are haunted by evil spirits and they usually avoid a visit to such places. Insanity, epilepsy, chest pain, etc., are generally considered the result of the attack of evil spirits.

Only magical medicine is effective in the treatment of these diseases. An able *Manthrakkaran* can diagnose the cause of such diseases and ward off the evil spirit from the patient through some magical rites. The assistance of benevolent gods is essential to ward off such evil spirits from the patients. After the warding off ceremony the *Manthrakkaran* will usually give the patient some amulets or talisman to wear on the body. This is a prophylactic measure to prevent attacks that may occur in future.

(d) Practice of Sorcery and Disease

The Muthuvans believe that, through sorcery a man can bring diseases to people. Through divination a *Manthrakkaran* can diagnose the cause of such diseases. The diseases originating from sorcery can be healed either through praying to the deities or by initiating proper counter magic to destroy the power of sorcery.

Society is not favourably disposed towards a sorcerer who is found indulging in it to harm others. He will be caught and brought before the council of elders. After trial, the elders will punish him, if found guilty. The usual punishment will be beating with a stick.

(e) Breach of Taboo and Disease

The Muthuvans observe certain taboos in their socio-religious life. Eating the meat of a cow or a buffalo is considered a taboo. Visiting or going near a menstrual hut also is a taboo. Such a person will be considered as polluted and he has to take bath before entering his house. Visiting a woman and a child, while they are living in the seclusion hut after confinement is a taboo. The Muthuvans consider their agricultural field and the area around the temples and jungle groves as divine. Defecating or urinating in such places is a taboo. Killing of dogs and cobras is another taboo. They hold that, one has to eat the flesh of a being which he killed, otherwise it is an offence.

Most of these taboos originated from religious beliefs. So the sanction of supernatural entities is behind these taboos. Consequently, the breach of a taboo will invite the wrath of gods and they will punish the human beings with diseases. Thus the occurrence of disease is directly related to the violation of taboo.

As the diseases caused due to the violation of taboo is supernatural in origin, no herbal medicine will be effective in checking them. Only the treatment of a *Manthrakkaran* will give relief to such a patient. Along with the performance of some magical rites, a number of offerings also will be made in the temples to please the deities.

(f) Yearning of leopard and disease

Some of the illnesses are caused due to the evil influences of wild beasts in the forests. To cite an example, a hungry leopard or tiger can influence the mental state of a man and turn him into a patient. Sometimes when a tiger or a leopard, sees a man in the wild forest, it wants to kill him to have a nice meal. Very often it may not be able to catch the man at that time. Then with an intense sense of yearning the beast will lick its left forelimb. It will think how nice it would have been, if he could catch that man.

Then onwards, that person will start showing insane behaviour. Occasionally he will shiver and suffer from acute fever. The shivering is supposed to occur whenever the leopard thinks about this man. Thus he is always under the control of the vicious desire of the leopard. At last, the person will go alone to the interior forest, like a somnambulist, and become a pray to the hungry leopard.

It is here that the services of the *Pulivathy* become essential. An able Pulivathy can save the patient from the leopard, if he is contacted in time. He can diagnose the disease and through adequate magical rites, can eradicate the vicious influence of the leopard. The yearning of the leopard will die down after the performance of the necessary warding off ceremonies by the *Vathy*. Afterwards he will tie an amulet on the person's upper arm which will guard him against the attack of wild beasts in future.

(g) Soul loss and disease

The Muthuvans believe that the evil spirits which haunt the thick of forests can inflict a number of maladies upon human beings. A demon can capture the soul of a man and hide it in a cave inside the forest. After losing the soul, the happiness and brightness on a person's face will vanish and he will be gloomy always. Gradually he will lose the strength of the body, and become a patient in a short while.

Through divination, an *Anthervathy* can diagnose the cause of this illness. Both herbal medicine and magic are used as remedies to check this illness. The assistance of the benevolent spirits also will be sought for controlling the evil demons. After performing the adequate magical rites, the *Anthervathy* will visit the interior area of forest and collect some powerful medicinal herbs. Then he will grind these herbs well and make a paste of them. A mark will be made on the forehead of the patient, using this herbal paste. This will be continued for three days. After making this mark on the forehead, the demon will bring back the soul and re-insert it in the patient's body. The demon cannot resist the power of this herbal mark and the magic performed along with it. With the return of the soul, the patient will regain his strength and vitality.

MAGIC AS MEDICINE

The Muthuvans have deep faith in the efficacy of magic in curing diseases. When somebody is sick, they will first contact the *Manthrakkaran* for help. He will diagnose the cause of the illness through divination. At the time of divination he will invoke the dead ancestors and gods, through appropriate spells and incantations. They will convey the cause and remedies of illness to the *Manthrakkaran* and he will treat the patient according to these directions.

According to a *Manthrakkaran* the four major and frequently occurring causes of illness are, anger of god, anger of ancestral spirits, breach of taboo and possession of evil spirits. In the divination process there are separate methods to find out these different causes of illness. At one time, the divination is aimed to find out the involvement of only one causative agent. If that agent is found innocent, then the divination process will be aimed at another cause. If one method reveals that anger of god is not the reason for the illness, then the *Manthrakkaran* will test whether the wrath of the ancestral spirit is the cause of the illness. So it is a trial and error method.

After divination the *Manthrakkaran* will advise the relatives of the patient to make some offerings in a certain temple of that locality. The shaman will also give the patient some herbal medicines which are very effective in checking the disease. The efficacy of herbal medicine will be increased through chanting some spells and treating them with certain magical rituals. If the medicine is very powerful and efficacious, then there is no need of performing magic to enhance its healing power. But some diseases like *asthma* need magic, while material medicine is taken for its cure.

DIVINATION METHODS

Through the divination the *Manthrakkaran* diagnoses the cause of disease and its possible remedies. This is the prior step taken before starting the treatment of a patient. It will give, him a clear picture of the disease, its nature, origin and possible methods of cure. The Muthuvans have more than one method of divination. However, in all types of divination, the assistance of the gods and ancestral spirits is essential for the shaman to diagnose a disease and to find out its remedies.

1. Olippu

Olippu is one method of divination applied for diagnosis and also for finding out the future strategy of treatment. For performing this magical ritual, the shaman will take a cane basket, known as *Olippukotta* and put a number of copper and bronze pieces into it. A shaman possesses a cloth bag, full of bronze and copper pieces, for this purpose. After putting the copper and bronze pieces into the *Olippukotta* he will start chanting spells and tinkle the basket. He will bend over the basket, while chanting the spells. First he will shake the basket very slowly and will gradually increase its momentum. When it reaches the climax, the jingling sound will be heard above the chanting of spells. This jingling sound and chanting of spells will create a special mood, which is ideal for inducing suggestions to the patient.

When the jingling attains the climax the shaman will be possessed by the ancestral gods and jungle spirits. So he will reach a trance state and his body will start shaking. Sometimes, he will dance in a wild fashion, holding the *Olippukotta* in his hands. First the dance will be at a slow pace and gradually he will increase the speed. At the climax of the dance, the *Manthrakkaran* will ask the ancestral gods about the reason for the occurrence of this disease and the possible remedies for it. Then the ancestral gods will reveal the cause and remedies of the disease to him. The shaman will tell these matters to the relatives of the patient. Afterwards, he will stop the dance and the tinkling of the basket and gradually return to his normal state of mind. The patient and his relatives will act according to the orders given by the *Manthrakkaran* for the healing of the illness. This will usually include taking of herbal medicines and giving offerings in the temple.

2. Kuri Veyppu

Another method of divination used for the diagnosis of disease is known as *Kuri Veyppu.* For divination purpose, the *Manthrakkaran* will take a winnowing basket and a pinch of paddy grains. Then he will invoke the ancestral spirits and jungle deities through chanting of spells. Only through their help he can reach correct conclusions. Then he will place the paddy grains in one corner of the winnowing basket and spread them by moving two grains each from the group. In the end, if two grains are left, then it indicates that there is some trouble in the relationship with the gods and they are angry with the patient. If only one paddy grain is left in the end, then it indicates that there is no problem in the relationship with the supernaturals. Then he will try to find out whether there is any attack of evil spirits.

The same process will be repeated to find out which god is behind the disease and what offering is needed to heal the patient. When moving the paddy grains the shaman will meditate that particular god. In the end if only one grain is left, then it can be assumed that there is no problem with that god. Then the shaman will meditate another god and repeat the process with the paddy grains. The offering needed to the gods also can be found out in the same way. When the divination is over, the *Manthrakkaran* will tell the patient, about his findings and the disease will be healed if the patient follows his directions.

HEALING RITUALS

The Muthuvans have a number of rituals connected with the treatment of various diseases. The rituals vary according to the nature of the illness. These healing rituals are generally put to use in the treatment of diseases due to supernatural causes. Therefore, only a *Manthrakkaran* or a *Vathy* can officiate at these rituals for the benefit of his patients. The rituals are employed in the treatment, always after the divination process. So each ritual will be conducted according to the nature of the disease causing agent.

Some of the rituals need the active participation of the patient while some others are conducted by the shaman himself. Sacrifices are a part of some of these healing rituals. In all these rituals, the shaman invokes the deities for their intervention in the matter. Actually the shaman will be possessed by their power on most of the occasions. The performance of these healing rituals will give much confidence to the patient. He will be happy that something is being done for the curing of his illness.

1. Magic for backache

There is a magical ritual to get rid of the back pain. If a person has backache or dislocation, the *Manthrakkaran* will first make him stand upright. Then he will take two slender, straight wooden or bamboo poles, of the same length and keep them above the hip region of the patient on both sides. Then the patient will be told to hold them firmly over his hip. The other ends of these four feet long poles will rest on the hands of another person, who will stand face to face with the patient. He will be told by the shaman to keep the poles parallel to the ground, in the same level.

After arranging the polls the *Manthrakkaran* will take some hot ash from the hearth. Then he will chant a number of spells to make the ash powerful. Through the spells he will also invoke the help of the ancestral spirits and gods to assist him to heal the pain of the patient. Then he will take a pinch of ash using the thumb and index finger of the right hand and sprinkle it slowly in the middle part of the poles. He will move his hand slowly forward and backward sprinkling the ash over both the poles. He will chant some spells in a low pitch while performing this ritual. This process will be repeated with four or five pinches of ash. The healing ritual will be over with the sprinkling of this ash. Then the poles will be removed and the patient will go back to his home.

Sometimes a few medicinal herbs will be given to him either to prepare a decoction and consume or to make a paste and apply over the region of pain.

2. Kozhiyae parappikal

This is a magical ritual conducted to ward off the evil spirits possessed in a patient. Such a person will be suffering from diseases like epilepsy, insanity, anemia and chest pain for a longtime due to the attack of evil spirits and devils. A *Manthrakkaran* can diagnose the cause of such prolonged illness by his divination techniques. He can find out which evil spirit or *Muni* is residing in the body of the patient.

After detecting the evil spirits, the shaman will order the relatives of the patient to bring a cock to him. A black cock is often preferred for this purpose. When the cock is brought, he will rotate it around the head of the patient, three times. He will chant a number of spells at this time and will be in a state of trance. After rotating the cock around the head, he will keep the head of the cock in touch with the forehead of the patient, for a few seconds. Then all the evil spirits and devils residing in the patient will enter the body of the cock. Thus the evil spirits will be captured in the body of the cock and the patient will be free from them. He will soon recover from his illness.

Afterwards, the *Manthrakkaran* will hold the cock in his hand and chant some spells looking on it, in order to assure that the evil spirits will not escape from the cock. Then he will go to the interior of forest and drive it away from the sight. Thus the evil spirits go away from the patient, while that cock flies away from him. Nobody will ever catch this cock or eat its flesh, lest the evil spirits would enter his body.

3. Thullal

Thullal is a very powerful and efficacious magical ritual performed to cure the diseases originating due to the possession of evil spirits and devils on a person. After the possession of evil spirits, that person will be affected by various diseases and will lose all his vigour to do any work. Ordinary medicine and magic will not bring any relief in such cases. Only through some powerful magical techniques can that person be healed and brought back to his former condition.

If somebody is suffering from an illness for a prolonged period and is not responsive to treatments, he will be taken to a *Anther Vathy*. Through divination he will diagnose the cause of the illness. If the illness is due to the possession of evil spirits, the *Vathy* will suggest to the relatives of the patient to conduct a warding off ceremony to drive out the evil spirits residing in the patient.

The warding off ceremony is always conducted during the night, in the courtyard of the patient's house. A particular place will be selected and cleaned using a broom. Then eighteen leaves of the *Channakuva* plant (Costus speciosus) are brought and spread on the ground. The leaves are arranged in a square pattern. Then five live torches made of reed pipe and coconut oil are brought and one is placed in the centre and others in the four corners of the square. If the patient is a female, then a cock and if the patient is a male, then a hen will be brought and placed near the square with its legs tied with a strand.

Afterwards, the *Vathy* will sit in one corner of the square and start chanting spells to invoke various supernatural spirits. A bowl containing turmeric water will be brought and kept by his side. Incences will be burned to impart a special mood to the whole atmosphere. Then the patient will be brought and made to sit opposite the *Vathy*. The chanting of spells will get increased momentum and sound, after the arrival of the patient. He will reach an ecstasy in a short time and his body will start trembling. Then his words become unintelligible and he will stand up and walk around the patient, three times. Each time, when he comes face to face with the patient, he will produce a *Khreem* sound and sprinkle the turmeric water over him. Then he will go back to his place, sit on the ground and resume the chanting of spells. After some time he will again come back and repeat the same process. This will be done at least six times. The *Khreem* sound is produced to threaten the evil spirits. The turmeric water is sprinkled to purify the body of the patient. After repeated sprinkling of the turmeric water, the patient will appear like one who has bathed in that solution.

Then the *Vathy* will take the fowl and move it three times in a circle above the head of the patient. While doing this, all the evil spirits and devils residing in the patient will leave him and enter that fowl. Then the fowl will be sacrificed by cutting away its head. The blood gushing out from the throat will be poured over a leaf. Three holes will be made on the leaf using a knife. So the blood will be drained away through those holes to the earth.

After sacrificing the fowl, the *Vathy* will lie down on a mat on the floor. Then his assistant will cover him with another mat. If he is not covered, the evil spirits and devils exorcized from the patient will enter his body and kill him. Only the tip of his hands and knife can be seen outside.

The meat of the fowl will be cooked by the assistant of the shaman and only elders are allowed to eat it. Since the fowl is used to ward off the evil spirits, its flesh is polluted. If the youngsters and children eat this meat, the evil spirits will enter their body.

Thullal is a very efficacious healing ritual and is utilized only as a last resort, in the case of serious and prolonged illness. If a patient could not be healed after performing this ceremony, no other medicine or magic can save him.

In the present age, only very few old *Vathykal* know how to conduct this ritual. There may be only one person in a whole area. So the people of the neighbouring hamlets will come to seek his help. Then he will go along with them and carry out the *Thullal* ceremony to heal the patient.

4. Dogbite and Snakebite

There is one magical treatment to heal the wound and remove the poison, resulting from a dogbite. For removing the poison a small reed pipe is placed over the wound and then the *Manthrakkaran* sucks the blood from the wound and spits away the poisoned blood entering his mouth. He chants spells before sucking the poison. After the flow of blood ceases, herbal medicine is applied on the wound.

The same process is followed in the case of snakebite. In this case there is no need for the reed pipe to touch the wound. It is believed that while chanting the spells the venom of the snake will automatically come out and enter the reed pipe. All the venom will be removed after performing this ritual two or three times.

SMALLPOX, CHICKENPOX AND MEASLES

These are the important diseases originating from the wrath of goddess *Mariyamma*. These diseases cannot be cured by taking material medicine. The condition of the patient will only become worse if medicine is given to him. *Mariyamma* will get more angry if medicine is taken to drive her out.

Therefore, no medicine will be given to the patient. But water made holy by the chanting of spells will be given to a patient suffering from the anger of *Mariyamma*. He has to take rest and avoid lying down near the fireplace. Diet control is the chief method to check these diseases. A patient must avoid eating hot rice, salt, chilly and side dishes prepared in oil. He can take only cold gruel and some vegetables prepared without using salt and oil. He cannot drink or bathe in cold water. By adhering to this special diet, and also through drinking the holy water, a patient can control his illness.

Special plates will be provided to the patient for taking food. The other members of the house also will have to adhere to some restrictions in the diet. In that house, the side dishes prepared by frying in oil and the seasoning of side dishes with oil and mustard seed shall be avoided. The smell of these food items will increase the anger of *Mariyamma* and thus aggravate the illness. The other members of the house will have to avoid frequent contact with the patient and he may lie down in one corner of the house, without being noticed by others. Only the members who nurse him should go near him. Such restrictions will prevent the spreading of the disease further.

For speedy relief, one has to pray to *Mariyamma* when suffering from the illness. This prayer is conducted in a special manner with the help of a *Manthrakkaran*. First, a little turmeric water will be taken in a shallow vessel and three or seven small flowers will be put in it. Then the *Manthrakkaran* will stand on his knees with folded hands and bend over the vessel containing the turmeric water. In this posture he will pray to *Mariyamma* to heal the patient by leaving him without causing more trouble. He will also make a vow, on behalf of the patient, that a cock will be sacrificed to *Mariyamma* during the next *Pongal* festival. The man who pray to *Mariyamma* must take bath before the ritual and his clothes also must be clean. The performer of this ceremony will tie a chisel on his neck with a black string.

ONION CHAIN AND MEASLES

When children are affected by measles or chickenpox, the parents will take either three, seven or nine onion bulbs and string them together into a chain. No spell will be chanted while preparing the chain, as chanting of spells will aggravate the wrath of *Mariyamma*. Then the onion chain will be put round the neck of the patient. The wearing of this chain will help to control the disease.

SMALL POX AND MAGIC

For reasons already stated, the Muthuvans will not resort to any magic or medicine when somebody is affected by smallpox, chickenpox or measles. However, if the disease attains the form of an epidemic and starts killing a number of people, then the *Vathykal* of the tribe will do some magical rituals to prevent the further spreading of the disease. Only an *Aakaya Vathy* belonging to the 'Melakuttom' clan can perform this ritual. *Mariyamma* herself is supposed to have given him power to control diseases like smallpox, chickenpox and measles.

As a preparation to perform this ritual, the *Aakaya Vathy* will bathe first and wear new clothes. Then he will smear sandalwood paste on his forehead. Afterwards he will wear a necklace comprising of the teeth and claws of a tiger, a leopard, a bear and a crocodile. This necklace possessing supernatural power, is known as *Uthrasimala*. It is a divine necklace, which is always kept in a wooden box. A *Vathy*, will wear it only to prevent the spreading of smallpox and also on the occasion of teaching magic to somebody.

After wearing this *Uthrasimala* the *Vathy* becomes very powerful. Then he can control even goddess *Mariyamma* who is responsible for the smallpox. When he invokes the goddess, she will come and possess him. Then the *Vathy* will ask her, why she is angry with the people and what is needed to appease her anger. Then the goddess will convey to him the reason for the outbreak of the epidemic and its possible remedy. Very often a cock or goat will be sacrificed after this magical ritual to appease goddess *Mariyamma*.

TALISMAN

A talisman known as *Thayam* in the Muthuvan dialect is usually prepared by a *Manthrakkaran*. This is a device to prevent the attack of evil spirits, sorcerers and wild animals. A special tube made of silver or steel and having a length of two inches, is available in the market, for preparing the talisman. A fine powder of medicinal plants available in the forest, will be filled in the tube. The leaves, roots and tender shoots of various medicinal plants are collected and dried in the sun and afterwards crushed using a stone, for preparing the medicinal powder. The shaman will enhance the power of the medicinal powder by chanting some spells, while it is being filled in the tube. The tube will be closed after inserting the medicinal powder and then tied on the upper arm or on the waist, using a black thread.

Neither an evil spirit, nor a sorcerer can attack a person who wears this talisman. So he will always be protected from such kind of diseases coming through these agents. It can also protect its wearer from the evil eye of a leopard or tiger. The power of a talisman will last till the death of its wearer.

There is also another method for the preparation of a talisman. In this method, the '*Manthrakkaran*' takes a small piece of copper sheet, which is very thin and flexible and inscribes on it certain magical formulae using an iron stiletto or nail. The magical formulae are very powerful and they can protect the wearer of the talisman, from the attack of evil spirits, sorcerers and wild animals. For preparing the talisman, the copper sheet inscribed with the magical formulae is rolled up and then inserted in a silver or steel tube. After closing the tube it is tied round the waist or on the upper arm. Only few people prepare talisman by this method, as it is more costly than the first one.

ILLNESS AND THERAPEUTIC RECIPES

In the following pages the names of all the common illnesses and the remedies employed by the medicinemen of the Muthuvan Community are given. The exact dosage and the quantity of ingredients required could not be given as the medicinemen are not in a position to specify this aspect. Both Malayalam and English names of the illnesses are provided. The names of medicinal plants are given in the Muthuvan dialect along with their botanical names. However, the botanical names of a few plants could not be found out even after much effort. So they are given as 'Unidentified' (UI) in brackets.

NAMES OF ILLNESSES AND THERAPEUTIC RECIPES

1. *Thalavedana* (Head ache)

a. Grind the leaves of *Kongini* (Lantana camara) and *Venappacha* (Blumea lacera) and smear this paste on the forehead.

b. Crush the seeds of *Neerpezhu* (Barringtonia acutangula) and pack them in a cloth. Use it as an inhalant.

c. Catch some *Kuzhiyana* (the ant lion) and grind them well to make a paste. Smear this paste on the forehead.

d. Grind some mustard seed and a few bulbs of *Veluthully* (Allium sativum) into a paste and smear it on the forehead.

e. Grind the bark of *Thanny* (Terminalia bellirica) and smear this paste on the forehead.

2. *Nenchuvedana* (Chest pain)

a. Crush the root of *Edana* (Olea dioica) and extract the juice and drink. Smear a part of it on the chest also.

b. Grind together the tender leaves of *Mungi* (Bambusa arundinacea), the rhizome of *Inchy* (Zingiber officianel) and a piece of jaggery to make a paste. Then boil a young chicken in water and extract a part of this solution and mix it with the paste and take.

c. Crush the bark of *Karana* (Aristolochia indica) and extract the juice and drink.

d. Grind together a piece of *Chandanam wood* (Santalum album), *Verukinpuzhu* (venter of Civet cat) and the leaves of *Mulachimullu* (Xanthoxylum rhetsa) and mix it with hot water and drink.

3. *Murivu* (Wound)

a. Collect the leaves of *Edampiri Valampiri* (Helicteres isora) and dry them. Pound these dried leaves thoroughly and apply the powder on the mouth of the wound.

b. Mash the leaves and tender stem of *Murikooty* (Zornja diphylla) and cover the wound with it. Tie with a piece of cloth to fix the medicine on the wound.

c. Grind soot and a piece of dry turmeric (Curcuma longa) and apply this powder on the wound.

d. Roast the seeds of *Kurumulaku* (Piper nigrum) and black *Thelly* (Canarium strictum) in coconut oil and grind them well. Take this powder in a dry cloth and apply this poultice over the wound.

e. Boil the tender leaves of *Nilapulladi* plant (UI) and the *Ottupullu* (Trlumfetta rhomboidea) in coconut oil. Extract this oil and apply on the wound.

f. The sap obtained from a *Vazha* plant (Musa paradisiaca) while cutting its inflorescence is applied on the wound.

4. *Theeppollal* (Burn)

a. Apply honey over the affected part of the body.

b. Grind the leaves of *Elamulachy* (Kalanchoe laciniata) and smear this paste on the affected part.

c. Mash the leaves of *Veppu* (Azadiracta indica) and pack in a cloth and apply as a poultice.

5. *Pani* (Fever)

a. Crush the leaves and roots of *Panikoorka*, (Coleus aromaticus) and drink the infusion.

b. Grind the leaves of *Thulasi* (Ocimum sanctum) dilute it with water and drink.

c. Roast *Ully* (Allium cepa) and the leaves of *Thulasi* (Ocimum sanctum) in coconut oil and afterwards grind them into a paste. Apply this paste on the head and take bath in hot water.

6. *Chuma* (Cough)

a. Collect the sap of *Palvally* (Ichnocarpus frutescens) and mix it with hot water and drink.

b. Prepare a decoction by boiling the seeds of *Kadukka* (Terminalia chebula), the rhizome of *Inchy* (Zingiber officianel) and *Pepper* (Piper nigrum) in water and drink.

c. Chew *Pepper* (Piper nigrum) and common salt (NaCl) and swallow the juice.

d. Drink the water found inside the shoot of *Elly* (Bambusa arundinacea) for three days.

7. *Nilankarichuma* (Whooping cough)

a. Roast the meat of bat in gingelly oil and eat.

b. Cook the meat and faeces of a white monkey and take.

8. *Kannilasukham* (Eye Disease)

a. Mash the tender leaves of *Kalthamara* (Hybanthus enneaspermus) and dilute it with water and filter through a cloth. Use this juice as an eye drop.

b. Crush the tender shoots of *Panal* (Glycosmis pentaphylla), *Vellila* (Mussaenda glabrata), *Kattumulla* (Jasminum angustifolium) and

Vettila (Piper betel) and extract the infusion. Afterwards mix it with honey and breast-milk and apply as an eye drop.

c. Boil the *Muyalcheviyan* (Emilia sonchifolia) in toto, in water and filter this solution through a cloth. After proper cooling use this solution as an eye drop.

9. *Vayarilakkam* (Dysentery)

a. Crush the bark of *Kottam* (Grewia microcos) and extract the juice and drink.

b. Grind the tuber of *Padathali* (Cyclea peltata) and dilute it with water and drink.

c. Mash the tuber of *Naruneendy* (Hemidesmus indicus) and drink the juice.

d. Drink the honey of small bees twice daily for three days.

e. Grind a piece of *Chandanam* wood (Santalum album) and make it a paste by mixing with water and drink.

f. Mash the stem of *Kattukodi* (Piper trioicum) and drink the juice.

g. Grind the dry seed of *Kattukamuku* (Pinanga dicksonii) and mix this powder with water and *drink*,

h. Mash the shoot and root of *Thondy* (Sterculia urens) and drink the juice.

i. Crush the northbound bark of *Nelly* (Emblica officinalis), the northbound bark of *Njaval* (Syzygium cumini) and the bark of *Kottam* (Grewia microcos) and extract the juice and drink.

10. *Vayarukadi* (Diarrhoea with defecation of blood)

a. Take, the root of *Perikilam* (Clerodendrum viscosum) with equal quantities of *Nilampala* (Euphorbia hirta) and *Muyalcheviyan* (Emilia sonchifolia) in toto and cook them with rice and eat.

b. Extract the gum of *Elavu* (Bombax ceiba) and boil in water with a little salt (Nacl) and drink.

c. Grind the seeds of *Kattuvazha* (Musa superba) and mix this powder in black tea and drink.

d. Prepare a decoction by boiling the seeds of *Kaduka* (Terminalia chebula) in water and drink in the morning. Drink a decoction made of the unripe fruits of *Vilarmaram* (Feronia limonia) at noon. Grind the leaves of *Kanchavu* (Cannabis sativa) and take at night. Continue this medicine for six days.

11. *Chory* (Scabies)

a. Extract the oil from the bark of *Poovam* (Schleichera oleosa) and apply on the scabies.

b. Grind the leaves of *Vathamveratti* (Artanema sesamoides) and apply this paste on the scabies.

c. Prepare a decoction by boiling the leaves of *Thumba* (Leucas zeylanica) and Karuka (Cynodon dactylon) in water and drink.

d. Boil the shoots of *Incha* (Acacia caesia) in a large quantity of water and bathe in this hot water.

12. *Puzhukady* (Ring-Worm)

a. Crush the root of *Therakam* (Ficus exasperata) and apply the juice on the affected part of the body.

b. Grind the leaves and tender stem of *Shatavari* (Asparagus recemosus) and smear this paste on the affected part of the body. This medicine is also very efficacious in healing the prickly heat.

13. *Krumikadi* (Pinworm)

a. Eat raw fruits of Kaplanga (Carica pappaya) daily in the morning, continuously for six days.

b. Boil the tender shoot of *Elly* (Bambusa arundinacea) in water and drink that solution.

14. *Virashalyam* (Tape-worm & Round-worm Infestation)

a. Prepare a decoction by boiling the leaves of *Muyalcheviyan* (Emilia sonchifolia) in water and drink.

b. For worm infestation among the children, grind a piece of *Vayambu* (Acorus calamus) and dilute with water, and drink.

15. *Pampukadi* (Snake bite)

a. Grind the leaves of *Ganja* (Cannabis sativa) with the fruit of *Cherunarakam* (Citrus aurantifolia) and apply this paste on the part where the snake bit. Take it inside also.

b. Grind the leaves and root of *Analivegam* (Alstonia venenata) and smear this paste on the wound.

c. Grind a piece of *Kasturimanjal* (Curcuma aromatica) and dissolve it in breast-milk and drink. Apply it also on the wound, especially for the bite of cobra.

d. Grind the root of *Garudakodi* (Aristolochia indica) and *Vayambu* (Acorus calamus) and take inside.

e. Drink a solution prepared by dissolving *turmeric* powder (Curcuma longa) in water. Then place, the chemical matter at the end of a match-stick, on the wound and ignite it. When that chemical substance burns, the poison also will burn along with it.

f. Grind together a piece of boar's tusk, old pepper (Piper nigrum), *Kattutheppali* (Piper longum) and *Veluthulli* (Allium sativum) and mix it with a little *Kadi* (sour gruel) to make it a paste. Then add some breast-milk to this medicine and place it on the head of the patient.

16. *Pattikadi* (Dog bite)

a. Grind the seeds of *Marotti* (Hydnocarpus pentandra) and apply this paste on the wound.

b. Grind the *Pattiche viyan (UI)* in toto and smear on the wound.

c. Crush an old earthern pot and grind the pieces into a powder and apply this powder on the wound.

17. *Vayaruvedana* (Belly pain)

a. Crush the bark of *Maruthu* (Terminalia paniculata) and add a little salt (NaCl) into the juice and drink.

b. Boil the leaves of *Puliyarila* (Oxalis corniculata) in water and drink this decoction.

c. Mash the fruits of *Nelly* (Emblica officinalis) and the bark of *Kottam* (Grewia microcos) and drink the infusion.

d. Grind the leaves of *Kariveppu* (Murraya koenigii) and the tuber of *Kacholam* (Campferia galanga) and dilute it with water and drink.

e. Chew a Vettila leaf (Piper betel) with a little soot and a few crystals of common salt (NaCl) and swallow the Juice.

18. *Palluvedana* (Tooth ache)

a. Boil the seeds of *Aanachunta* (Solanum stramoniifolium) in water and gargle the mouth with this warm solution.

b. Grind the bark of *Karilavu* (Lannea coromandelica) and smear this paste on the gums.

c. Boil the seeds of *Mullichedy* (Carissa spinarum) in the oil extracted from *Veppu* (Azadiracta indica). Then bend over this vessal, open the mouth and receive the vapour emitting from it into the mouth.

19. *Manjapitham* (Jaundice)

a. Grind the tender shoots of *Aavanakku* (Ricinus communis), *Aadalotakam* (Adathoda vasica) and the dry rhizome of *Manjal* (Curcuma longa) and mix it with the infusion obtained by crushing the leaves of *Nilappana* (Curculigo orchioides). Take this mixture three times a day.

b. Crush the dried *Verukinpuzhu* (venter of Civet cat) and boil it in water and drink.

c. Mash the bark of *Manjakadampu* (Haldina cordifolia) and drink the juice.

d. Prepare a decoction by boiling *Kizhanelly* (Phyllanthus fraternus) in toto, in water and drink.

e. Grind the northbound root of *Panthalavira (UI)* and mix it with goat's milk. Then put a few red hot pebbles into it and drink this mixture while it is hot.

20. *Apasmaram* (Epilepsy)

a. Crush the root of *Kamalu* (Flemingia strobilifera) and prepare a decoction by boiling it in water and drink.

b. Prepare a decoction by boiling the bark and root of *Aamathali* (Trema orientalis) and *Cherupulladi* (Indigofera linnaei) in water and drink for one month.

21. *Shwasammuttal* (Asthma)

a. Crush the northbound bark of *Arampuli* (Piliostigma malabaricum) and extract the juice by filtering through a cloth. Take it for one week. Avoid taking bath while using this medicine.

b. Prepare a decoction by boiling the leaves of *Parppadakapullu* (Oldenlandia corimbosa) in water and drink.

c. For children, eating the cooked meat of white monkey is very efficacious to check asthma.

22. *Kushtam* (Leprosy)

a. Grind the bark of *Aattuvanchy* (Humboldtia vahliana) and *Karilavu* (Lannea coromandelica) with the fruits of *Kakamthodi* (Trichosanthes tricuspidata) and smear this paste over the affected portion of the body.

b. Crush the fruits of *Pazhamunpala* (Manilkara hexandra) and *Karimkottakodi* (UI) and extract the juice and drink.

23. *Neeru* (Oedima)

a. Grind *Muyalcheviyan* (Emilia sonchifolia) in toto and smear this paste on the body.

b. Grind the leaves of *Ganja* (Cannabis sativa), root of *Elantha* (Ziziphus mauritiana) and the bulbs of *Chuvannully* (Allium cepa) and apply this paste on the body. This is more effective in curing the oedima on the legs.

24. *Vatham* (Rheumatism)

a. Extract oil from the seeds of *Odal* (Sarcostigma kleinii) and smear on the body.

b. Grind the roots of *Ooram* (Urena lobata) and apply this paste on the body.

c. Grind the leaves of *Vetty* (Aporusa *lindleyana*) and massage the body with this paste.

d. Mash the leaves and tender stem of *Vathakoduveli* (UI) and the bark of Palakapaiyani (Oroxylum indicum) and pack them, in a cloth. Then apply this poultice on the affected part of the body.

e. Make some live coal by burning dry coconut shells and spread the leaves of *Erukku*

(Calotropis gigantia) over it. Then allow the patient to lie over it to cure back ache.

25. *Ulukku* (Sprain)

a. Grind the leaves of *Nilamparanda* (Desmodium triflorum) and smear this paste on the affected part of the body. Also give a steam bath to the aching part.

b. Grind the *Nilappana* (Curculigo orchioides) in toto and apply this paste on the aching portion of the body.

c. Warm the leaves of *Nayoori* (*UI*) and with that give a hot massage over the aching part of the body.

26. *Chathavu* (Bruise)

a. Cook the bark of *Venga* (Pterocarpus marsupium) with broken rice and take this gruel.

27. *Bone* Setting

a. Smear the fat of either *Malampampu* (Python) or *Cherapampu* (the Rat-Snake) on the broken limb. Give a bandage with fresh cloth and with straight bamboo splints. Change the bandage and apply the above medicine on alternate days.

b. Grind the root of *Pannikizhangu* (Pueraria tuberosa) along with a hen's egg and apply this paste after setting right the broken limb. Then cover that portion of the body with the wet *payal* (water plants like green algae) from river and secure with two. pieces of bamboo splints. Change the bandage and apply the above medicine on alternate days for a month.

28. *Vayu* (Gas trouble)

a. Roast a *Vattalmulaku* (Capsicum sp) by placing it over the burning coals and grind it along with soot and common salt (NaCl) and take.

b. Crush the rhizome of *Inchy* (Zingiber officianel) along with the seeds of *Kurumulaku* (Piper nigrum) and *Kattutheppoly* (Piper longum) and prepare a decoction by boiling it in water and drink.

29. *Schardy* (Vomiting)

a. Mash a piece of the rhizome of *Inchy* (Zingiber officianel) and drink the juice.

b. Eat the green leaves of *Kariveppu* (Murraya koenigii) in the raw form.

30. *Constipation*

a. Mash the root of *Adam Hawa* (Vinca rosea) and prepare a decoction by boiling it in water and drink.

31. *Arshasu (Piles)*

a. Prepare a decoction by boiling the bark, flowerbuds and tender root of *Peral* (Ficus bengalensis) in water and drink.

b. Grind the ripe seeds of *Paval* (Momordica charantia) and smear this paste on the anus.

c. Take a *Chuvannully* (Allium cepa) and put a few incisions on it with a knife and keep it in the rectum while going to sleep at night.

d. Mash the *Puliyarila* (Oxalis corniculata) in toto and drink the infusion.

e. Prepare a decoction by boiling the seeds of *Kadukka* (Terminalia chebula) and a piece of dried rhizome of *Manjal* (Curcuma longa) in water and drink.

32. *Thondaveekam* (Tonsilitis)

a. Mash the leaves of *Muyalcheviyan* (Emilia sonchifolia) along with common salt (NaCl) and *Ully* (Allium cepa) and extract the juice. Smear this juice inside the throat and also apply it on the head. Continue this for three days in the morning and in the evening.

33. *Vayilkuru* (Boil in the Mouth)

a. Eat the ripe fruits of *Manathakkali* (Solanum nigrum)

b. Grind together the leaves of *Kudakan* (Centella asiatica), the rhizome of *Manjal* (Curcuma longa) and the seeds of Kurumulaku (Piper nigrum) and take this paste.

34. *Chevi Vedana* (Ear ache)

a. Crush the bark of *Idampiri Valampiri* (Helicteres isora) and extract the juice. Use this juice as an ear-drop.

b. Mash the leaves of *Kattupadavalam* (Trichosanthes cucumerina) and extract the infusion, and use it as an ear-drop.

35. *Raktham pokku* (Bleeding of women)

a. Grind the leaves of *Aattuvanchi* (Humboldtia vahliana), dilute it with water and drink.

36. To check the problems at the time of Delivery

a. Mash the tender stem of *Vellila* (Mussaenda glabrata) with the bark of *Thekku* (Tectona grandis) and extract the juice by filtering through a cloth. Give it to the pregnant woman to drink.

b. Grind the tender shoots of *Chudali* (*UI*) and smear this paste on the abdominal portion of a pregnant woman.

c. Prepare a decoction by boiling the leaves of *Unnam* (Grewia tilifolia), *Thottavady* (Mimosa pudica), *Kurumthotti* (Sida acuta) and the seeds of *Kanjiram* (Strychnos nux-vomica) in water, and allow the pregnant woman to drink it.

37. Contraceptive for Women

a. Grind the roots of *Balankuravan* (*UI*) and mix it with little water and drink. Take this continuously for one month. Then that woman will not become pregnant for one Year. Repeat the medicine after one year if that woman want to avoid further pregnancy.

b. Crush the roots of *Chukakala* (*UI*) and drink the juice to avoid pregnancy. If the woman want to give birth to a child in future, she has to drink a decoction prepared from the leaves of the same plant. Then she will become fertile.

38. For the Increased Production of Breast-milk

a. Crush the bark of *Mayilellu* (Vitex leucoxylon) and extract the infusion. Mix this with water and cook rice in that solution. Eat this rice for the increased production of breast-milk among lactating mothers.

39. *Moothram Chudil* (Inflammation of the Urethra)

a. Crush the seeds of *Kalluvazha* (Musa superba) and prepare a decoction by boiling it in water and drink.

b. Prepare a decoction by boiling the crushed roots of *Naruneendy* (Hemidesmus indicus) in cow's milk and drink.

40. *Ushnam* (Venereal Diseases)

a. Prepare a decoction by boiling the dried seeds of *Njeringil* (Tribulus terrestris) in water and drink.

b. Prepare a decoction from the root of *Chemparavally* (Ampelocissus arnottiana) and drink.

c. Prepare a decoction by boiling the root of *Nilappana* (Curculigo orchioides) in cow's milk and drink.

d. Mash the fruits and root of *Kattupoovarasu* (Thespesia lampas) and prepare a decoction by boiling it in water and drink.

Usually all these medicines which are effective in curing the venereal diseases, have to be taken continuously for long periods, sometimes even for several months.

41. *Thalamudipozhichil* (Falling of hair)

a. Boil the faeces of Bear in coconut oil and extract the oil by filtering through a cloth and apply it on the head.

42. *Paruvu* (Abscess)

a. Grind the rhizome of *Chembu* (Colacasia sp), which grows in the cavities of tree trunks, with a little unboiled rice and apply this paste on the abscess.

43. *Kalvedichkeeral* (Cracks in the feet)

a. Grind the fruits of *Champakam* (Michelia champaca) and apply this paste on the feet.

b. Grind the fruit of *Peral* (Ficus bengalensis) with its sap obtained from the bark, and apply this paste on the feet.

44. *Tharan* (Dandruff)

a. Mash *Orilathamara* (Ayonidium fruticosm) in toto and apply on the head as a shampoo.

b. Grind the leaves of *Uzhinja* (Cardiospermum halicacabum) and mix it in water. Use this solution as a shampoo.

Ethnomedicine and Change

The Muthuvans living in hamlets situated in the interior areas of forests like *Plamala, Variyam, Edamalakudy* etc. have very little contact with the people living in the outer world and want to preserve their traditional qualities intact. Generally, they depend upon ethnomedicine for checking the illnesses afflicting them. In such remote areas there are neither hospitals, nor any roads to bring the patients to the nearest hospital. So they have very few options, and fight against diseases in their traditional, primitive manner. For them ethnomedicine is more important and useful, than modern medicine.

However, they have admitted that, they will take a patient to hospital as a last resort, in case of serious ailments. Before taking a patient to any hospital, they will try all their traditional methods to cure the illness. When the patient seems to be in a critical condition, he will be taken to the nearest hospital. So he will reach the hospital in a worse stage and often modern medicine will be helpless to save that patient. This makes them feel that the hospitals cannot save patients. The death of the patient will be considered as the result of the inefficacy of modern medicine and not because of negligence in the early part of illness. Naturally, they hold the opinion that hospitals are places where a patient can die and it is useless to take anybody there for treatment.

The confidence in ethnomedicine is another major factor discouraging the Muthuvans from going to the hospitals. They believe that their traditional system of medicine can deliver them from all illnesses. It is easily available and also economical. They also believe that there is no effective medicine for certain categories of diseases like smallpox and chickenpox, which are supposed to be originating from supernatural causes.

So they are very reluctant to take the patients to hospitals. Sometimes, even in serious cases they may keep the patient in his house because even if they take the patient to a hospital chances of his recovery are very remote. Then they have to bring the dead body back home for burial. This is an uphill task when considering the nature of their terrain. To avoid this trouble, they keep the patients in their houses and treat them with their own ethnomedicine. There are no roads or good paths to reach their hamlets. So the non-availability of modern medicine helps them to maintain the status quo.

The Muthuvans living in the fringe areas of forests have some contact with the non-tribals and the welfare programmes of the government and voluntary agencies. The interaction with these people and their programmes motivate the Muthuvans to use modern medicine. The free and easy availability of modern medicine also persuades them to use it to check the diseases afflicting them. However, it is worth noting that even when they are exploiting the modern medical facilities they depend upon their ethnomedicine in order to get a complete cure. They believe that without the help of supernaturals the treatment will not give any favourable result to the patient. Thus modern medicine has only a complementary role along with ethnomedicine in the treatment of diseases even among the Muthuvans who live in the fringe areas of forests.

THE MANNANS

Like the Muthuvans, the Mannans also possess an ethnomedical system to combat the illnesses afflicting them. The use of various medicinal plants and the manipulation of supernatural forces through magical techniques are the two major parts of ethnomedicine of the Mannans. Ethnomedicine is influenced by other spheres of life like religion, morality, social values, economy, subsistence pattern, social mobility, etc. This system of medicine always functions to ensure the health and well-being of the members of the Community.

THE VICHAKARAN-HIS STATUS AND ROLE

The *Vichakkaran* is the most important functionary in the ethnomedical system of the Mannans. He can be equated to a shaman found in the traditional anthropological literature. The term *Vicha* may be a crude form of the Malayalam word *Vidya* which means knowledge, and *Karan* means one who possesses something. So the term *Vichakkaran* means one who possesses knowledge. In this context, knowledge denotes expertise in the art of shamanism. Also a *Vichakkaran* will have a good knowledge of the properties of various medicinal plants. He treats the patients mainly with the help of magical techniques. So his treatment is more symbolic and expressive. He may give some herbal remedies also to his patients, where it is necessary. As he possesses enormous knowledge in spells, magical rituals and in the qualities of medicinal herbs, other members of the community respect him. However, his social status is below that of the headman or *Kani*. In some hamlets like *Thalumkandam*, the headman functions also as a *Vichakkaran*. The *Vichakkaran* is not a full-time specialist, but lives like any other ordinary member of the community. He receives no remuneration for his service.

Any member of the community can approach him at any time, if he is suffering from an illness. It is the duty of the *Vichakkaran* to help him and relieve his trouble through his magic and medicine. People have strong faith in his capabilities and they follow his directions to get rid of the diseases. Thus a *Vichakkaran* helps the people to lead a happy life by rescuing them from the clutches of disease.

Divination is the usual method adopted by a *Vichakkaran* to diagnose a disease. This process is known as *Kodanki* and is undertaken with the help of magical spells and techniques. The assistance of supernatural forces is essential for all the steps in the divination and treatment of a *Vichakkaran*. Through divination he will find out the cause of the illness. The next step is treatment. This will depend upon the nature of the causal agent. For diseases originating from natural causes, he will prepare a herbal decoction and give it to the patient as medicine. Diseases due to supernatural causes will be dealt with by special magical means. Sometimes, he will advise the patients to wear a talisman or an amulet as a prophylactic measure. He knows how to prepare them.

THE VAIDYAN

Besides the *Vichakkaran* a *Vaidyan* will be present in many of the Mannan hamlets. He is a herbalist and possesses vast knowledge about various medicinal plants. He also knows how to make a number of medicinal preparations from various plants. But he has no special knowledge in shamanism and never employs magic to heal his patients. So he can cure only diseases originating from natural causes.

The *Vaidyan* has only a lower status than a *Vichakkaran*. He is not a full-time medicineman and his profession may not be the treatment of diseases. Rather, he is an ordinary member of the community who has a lot of knowledge about the qualities of various medicinal plants. There are no specialists among them. All of them deal with every kind of disease. His service is free. He is available always and is ready to visit the houses of patients whenever needed.

INITIATION OF A VICHAKKARAN

The initiation of a *Vichakkaran* is an important matter in the community life of the Mannans, as he has to play an important role in the well-being of the members of the community. The character and behaviour of a man who is to be trained as a *Vichakkaran* will be kept under observation for a certain period, before teaching him magic. Only an honest and sincere man with well balanced emotions will be taught magic.

There is no strict rule of inheritance in passing *Vicha* or the knowledge of magic, from one *Vichakkaran* to a new person. The novice must be an honest and sincere man with genuine interest in learning *Vicha*. Usually a nephew will be given preference to a son. A nephew is preferred because, he is a member of the same clan of the *Vichakkaran*. So when a nephew is taught, the *Vicha* will not pass outside the clan.

Before starting the study of magic, a potential learner will have a number of dreams. He will dream of a number of fantastic things, even during day time. Then this man will usually approach a *Vichakkaran* and tell him about the dreams and his desire to learn magic. Therefore, the frequent occurrence of dreams is considered as a sign of a potential learner of magic.

Vicha can be taught to a man at the age of 18 or 20 years. Actually age is not an important criterion in the teaching of the *Vicha*. The teacher must be satisfied with the capabilities of the student. The teacher will satisfy himself that the student will be able to grasp the various techniques and spells of the art of shamanism.

Before initiation, the student has to take an oath before the teacher: that he will use his *Vicha* only for the benefit of the community; he will not harm anybody through sorcery; he will protect the members of the community from diseases and other calamities; he will consider all the households as one and will work for the welfare of everybody; he will consider all the hearths and pots of the hamlet as one and will use his efforts to protect them. Then the teacher will advise the student thus: 'You must be honest in your words and deeds; you must not be carried away by anger or emotions; you must always seek satisfaction and well-being of others in preference to yours; you should not be happy when a fellow member is suffering; you should consider the fellow members as your brethren and it is your duty to work for the welfare of the community.'

The teaching generally takes place during night, when other members of the household are in sound sleep. The *Vicha* can be taught in daytime also. But there must not be anybody else present in the house. Another venue for teaching is the forest, often during an expedition to collect forest produces. In the forest, there is nobody to overhear what the teacher is saying and the student must be alone at the time of teaching.

After learning *Vicha*, a man should not harm another one through magic, even if some provocation came from the other side. One should not be arrogant since he knows *Vicha*. Instead he must be humble and willing to serve others in their need.

ATTAINING 'VICHA' FROM A DEAD TEACHER

Most of the *Vichakkaranmar* are very reluctant in revealing all the secrets of magic to their disciples. A *Vichakkaran* will conceal some of the important techniques from his disciples in order to maintain his superiority. Sometimes he will reveal these spells just before his death. If he could not do that, he will disclose the name of one of his disciples to whom he wants to give all his magical powers after his death. Then, through a magical ritual, that man can achieve *Vicha* from his teacher after his death. The method is more or less identical with that prevalent among the Muthuvans.

When this disciple performs some magical ritual in future, he will first invoke his teacher. Then the spirit of the teacher will come and sit upon the shoulder of his student. He can feel the weight of the spirit on his shoulder. But nobody else present there can see the spirit. As the magical ritual progresses the student will be possessed by the spirit of his teacher. Thus through the body of his student the dead *Vichakkaran* is performing the magical rite there. Assistance of the dead teacher is a great advantage for the student.

REMUNERATION OF 'VICHAKKARAN'

The *Vichakkaran* is not supposed to be paid for his services either in cash or in kind after he heals the illness of a patient through his magical treatment. He will never demand anything from the patient. But the patient can give some presents to the *Vichakkaran* to show his gratitude. It is the duty of a *Vichakkaran* to heal the diseases of people without any reward.

THE 'VATHY'

Vathy is a superior status attained by a *Vichakkaran* through achieving enormous knowledge and experience in the art of shamanism. Each *Vathy* needs a specialized knowledge in a particular branch of shamanism. Only by attaining old age and enough experience in the treatment of patients will a *Vichakkaran* be elevated to this high office. It is the *Raja Mannan* who officially gives the title of *Vathy* to a *Vichakkaran* after considering his knowledge and ability in the art of shamanism.

The *Vathy* has a superior status in the community and everybody has a feeling of awe and respect towards him. He looks after the well-being of the community by protecting it from the attack of diseases, evil spirits and wild beasts. Still he also lives like other ordinary members of the community and earn his livelihood by working in the soil and is not a full-time specialist.

Mainly there are five *Vathykal* (Pl.) in each hamlet to look after the affairs of the people living there. They are the *Aana Vathy*, *Puli Vathy*, *Adipisha Vathy*, *Edassary Vathy* and *Nadukuda Vathy*. These five *Vathykal* are specialists in different areas. *Aana Vathy* prevents the attack of wild elephants, while *Puli Vathy* protects the people from the attack of tigers and leopards. *Adipisha Vathy* checks smallpox and other diseases affecting the people. *Edassary Vathy* saves the people from the attack of evil spirits and demons. The *Nadukuda Vathy* is the leader of all the four *Vathykal*. He is not a specialist but he co-ordinates the activities of all these four specialist *Vathykal*. He belongs to the *Rajakkatt Ailavan* clan, while *Adipisha Vathy* and *Edassery Vathy* belong to the *Thekkida Ailavan* clan. *Aanavathy* belongs to the *Adukad Nagamalayan* clan, and the *Puli Vathy* belongs to the *Chalukapattu Urukaran* clan.

When a *Vathy* dies, usually his nephew will be selected as his descendant, to protect the members of the hamlet from calamities. The elders of the hamlet select a new *Vathy* on the 7th day after the demise of the old *Vathy*. But the relationship with the dead *Vathy* is not the chief criterion for the selection of his descendant. The major qualification which is considered for the selection of a *Vathy* is the knowledge in *Vicha*. There is no meaning in the selection of a person as a *Vathy* who doesnot possess any *Vicha*. Only through *Vicha* can a *Vathy* protect a hamlet from the attack of wild animals, evil spirits and diseases.

When a *Vathy* dies, people of the hamlet feel unsafe, because, he is responsible for the protection of the hamlet from all calamities. After his death, the magical fence which protects them will no more exists and they are exposed to all sorts of dangers. So they try to find out a new *Vathy* to fill the gap, and they also depend upon him for the protection of the hamlet in future.

If a suitable person cannot be found out on the 7th day after the demise of the old *Vathy* the elders will postpone the selection for one year.

Usually they will find out a new *Vathy* on the first death anniversary of the old one. For this one year, another senior *Vathy* of the hamlet will take over the additional duty of the dead one viz. protection of the hamlet in all ways.

THE MYTH OF 'PONNUM PUJARI'

Ponnum Pujari is the mythological high priest of the Mannan community. *Ponnum Pujari* means 'beloved priest' in Malayalam. He belongs to the *Rajakkattu Ailavan* clan of the *Aravakudy* phratry, which is the most superior clan. *Ponnum Pujari* is a mythological figure, who possesses super-human powers. It is believed that god gave him all these supernatural powers and he utilizes these divine qualities for the well-being of the entire humanity. He prays for the welfare and happiness of all sections of people, irrespective of their caste, creed, race, religion etc.

The Mannans believe that *Ponnum Pujari* holds a divine mirror in his right palm. He can watch the people living anywhere in the world, through this mirror. Thus he can see whether the people are living happily or are suffering from any diseases or other calamities.

The *Ponnum Pujari* presides over all the five *Vathykal*. When *Ponnum Pujari* learns from his divine mirror, that some calamity is going to occur in the world, he will relate this news to the *Vathykal*. It is then the duty of the *Vathykal* to protect the people from that danger. The *Vathykal* protect the Mannans and other tribal people from diseases, attack of wild animals and evil spirits by constructing magical fences around the area where they are living. Their fence is known as *Peruveli* which means a big fence. This functions as a device which guards the people from all the evil forces and diseases. It is believed that they construct this fence from sea to sea covering the whole earth wherever people live. After its construction no evil force can get inside its territory. The forces trying to trespass the fence will be destroyed by the magical power. This is the ultimate safety device under which the Mannans and all other people will be safe.

The *Vathykal* construct this fence through magical and superhuman powers. First the *Aanavathy* constructs his fence in the outermost side. Then the other three *Vathykal* also construct their own fences in the interior side of the first fence. The *Nadukuda Vathy* supervises and coordinates the construction of these fences. This fence which seals the members of the hamlet from outside influences prevents the diseases from affecting the people. Thus it can be rightly called a magical prophylactic device evolved by the *Vathykal*.

If any misfortune occurs among the Mannans, the *Ponnum Pujari* will summon the *Vathykal* and ask them to give the explanation for it as it is their duty to protect the people from all calamities. According to the Mannan mythology the *Ponnum Pujari* is selected by god himself. At present there is no *Ponnum Pujari* in the Mannan community. They believe that, if a new *Ponnum Pujari* is to be born, he has to be conceived by a virgin from among the goddesses.

Since there is no *Ponnum Pujari* at present, the *Vathykal* are not getting the information about the calamities occurring in the world. So they are not in a position to prevent the mishaps and protect the people. The Mannans believe that a new *Ponnum Pujari* will come in the near future to redeem them.

COMMON CONCEPTS OF ETIOLOGY

The Mannans identify both natural and supernatural causes for the occurrence of diseases. The common natural causes are poor diet, polluted food, over work, hostile climatic conditions, accidents, unhygienic surroundings, poor sanitary facilities, etc. The supernatural causes are more prominent and noticeable. They include sorcery, evil eye, attack of evil spirits, magical poison, anger of ancestral spirits, wrath of god, breach of taboo, curse of elders etc. The Mannans classify the diseases, according to the nature of the causal agent. The nature of treatment also depend upon the etiology.

However, after the contact with the modern civilization, certain new diseases are occurring among them. The Mannans do not know the actual cause behind these new diseases. So they have no adequate technique or medicine for the treatment of these modern diseases. Often they depend upon modern medicine for them. However, they continue to utilize ethnomedicine for diseases originating from supernatural causes.

NATURAL CAUSES OF DISEASE

1. Diet and Disease

The Mannans observe that the occurrence of disease was very few in the past, when they were following the occupation of shifting cultivation. Their own herbal remedies were effective in checking the few diseases that occurred. In present age, a number of diseases are affecting the people and traditional medicine is helpless to control them. The Mannans believe that, the changes that took place in the quality of diet is the main reason for the occurrence of new diseases. In former times, their diet consisted mainly of tubers, fruits, fresh vegetables, green leaves, honey, rats, fish, crabs, tortoises, monkeys, deers and so many other small games. They have also cultivated ragi and paddy in the forest.

Due to deforestation there are practically no animal's in the forest. The new encroachers ruthlessly killed them using guns. The present diet of the Mannans consists of rice, tapioca, ragi and other food items purchased from the market and from ration shops. Most of these food articles are less nutritious and adulterated. So they adversely affect the health of the Mannans. The deterioration of health due to change in the diet paves the way for occurrence of disease on a large scale.

2. Over work and insufficient food

Excessive work and inadequate intake of food are also reasons affecting the health of Mannans. Often, they have to engage in hardwork for their survival in the hostile terrains of their habitat. But after they have started the sedentary life-style, the variety of their diet has decreased largely. As a result of deforestation and over exploitation they are not getting many of the traditional food items obtained from the forest. The food available for them, now is less nutritious and chiefly contains starch. So the lack of a balanced diet plays a complementary role with the excessive work, in the deterioration of health.

3. CLIMATIC CONDITIONS

The Mannans lead their life facing the vagaries of a hostile climate. As their hamlets are situated in forests on hilly terrains, they are troubled by wind, rain and severe cold. In some places, during rainy season, the flooded forest rivers cut off all their connections with the outer world. Often they have to face starvation in such periods. The manual labourers will not get any work during rainy season and their family members will suffer due to lack of food. During summer, while working in the fields, they have to suffer the scorching heat of the sun. All these climatic conditions have a telling effect on their health. Consequently, they are more susceptible to diseases, especially during the lean season, when they are very weak due to lack of sufficient food.

4. POOR SANITATION

The sanitary conditions are not satisfactory in the Mannan hamlets. They have no latrines and all of them defecate in the open ground, which causes soil pollution. They use the river water for ablution and take drinking water from the same source. This contaminated water paves the way for the spreading of water borne diseases. The surroundings of Mannan households are not very hygienic and they have no safe method for the disposal of waste. The waste water from the kitchen often forms small ditches in the close vicinity of the dwelling places, which are ideal breeding grounds for mosquitoes. The solid wastes scattered around the houses attract the houseflies in large numbers. These unhygienic surroundings pave the way for the outbreak of diseases.

5. Modern Medicine and Disease

The Mannans claim that the changes occurred in the medical practice also play a role in the origin of new diseases. In the past they used to treat diseases with their own herbal remedies and magic. These herbal medicines were not harmful to the body but increased its vitality. Now a days they are using a number of modern medicines for the treatment of diseases. They believe that even though the modern medicines give quick relief for the illness they have a number of harmful effects to the body. Traces of modern medicine remain in the body for a long time and cause new disease. So the medicine used to recover from a disease, again functions as a causal agent for the origin of another disease.

SUPERNATURAL CAUSES OF DISEASE

The people are also concerned about the supernatural causes of disease. Some diseases diagnosed as originating from natural causes, will be considered as supernatural in origin, if they are not responding to any treatment for a long time. Through divination, a *Vichakkaran* can find out the cause of an illness. Treatment by employing magical rituals, offerings to deities, sacrifices, etc. are resorted to heal the supernatural diseases. For some particular diseases, herbal remedies also will be given after the magical treatment is over. But little importance is given to this material medicine, when compared to the magical rituals performed.

a. Sorcery and disease

Sorcery is a rare phenomenon among the Mannans. They consider sorcery as evil and before learning magic, one has to swear before his teacher, that he will not practise sorcery. But some wicked men may break this oath, and manipulate his magical powers to harm his brethren.

A sorcerer can cause disease to another person through the manipulation of evil forces. The diseases caused due to sorcery will last for a long time and will not respond to any ordinary treatment. Anemia, lack of appetite, dysentery, etc. are some of the symptoms of diseases caused by sorcery.

Seeking the help of god through prayer, is the best method to escape from the harmful effects of sorcery. Some offerings also must be made in the temple to please the god. Invoking his household deity and ancestral spirits also will be helpful. Then god will catch the sorcerer and punish him with various calamities. His punishment of the sorcerer will continue till he withdraws all his sorcery from his victim. Often the sorcerer will come to the man, whom he tried to destroy, and beg his pardon. If the man forgives the sorcerer then the anger of god will immediately disappear.

There is a social stigma against the practice of sorcery. Society usually isolates a sorcerer and nobody will co-operate with him or with his family members. Nobody will offer him food or water during his last days and he will meet with a tragic end. There will not be any prosperity in his house, as everybody's curse works against him.

The *Panchayat* of the Mannan community has its own method of trial and punishment of a sorcerer. If somebody is found performing sorcery, he will be caught and brought before the *Panchayat*. There he will be tied on to a pillar of *Murikku* tree (Erythrina indica). If the culprit did not confess the crime before the elders, people will gather firewood around the pole and burn it. After the confession he will be untied and then beaten on the thigh with a cane six, twelve, twenty four or thirty six times according to the seriousness of the crime. Then the *Kani* will ask him whether he will repeat his sorcery. The culprit has to take a vow before the council of elders that he will not repeat the same. He will swear this by the eight hundred jungle gods and the *Palkodi* which is the symbol of the community. With this the punishment will be over.

After receiving punishment the sorcerer should not show any uneasiness towards anybody in the hamlet and is supposed to co-operate with others. If he shows any enemity towards others, nobody will co-operate with him and in due course of time he will be excommunicated.

b. Evil Spirits and Disease

Some of the supernatural beings are malevolent by nature. They will cause various hardships to human beings by means of diseases, crop failures, attack of wild animals, accidents etc. Often they may indulge in such activities without any provocation from people. The attack of these evil spirits can be averted with the help of benevolent gods and also through some magical means.

Muni is one of the important evil spirits causing a lot of hardships to the people. Sometimes he will possess the body of a pregnant woman and suck the blood of the foetus and abort the pregnancy. The *Muni* can attack a person of any age and sex. A person susceptible to the attack of *Muni* will see a lot of bad dreams. He may dream that he is being trampled by an elephant, or is falling down from a mountain peak etc. After being possessed by the *Muni*, occasionally, the person will fall down on the ground with a foaming mouth. He will utter many things in unintelligible voice and roll and beat his head, hands and legs on the ground. In this struggle, he may sometimes hurt himself.

A *Vichakkaran* can rescue the person from the attack of *Muni*. He will invoke some benevolent deities for warding off the *Muni*. After being possessed by these deities he will construct a magical net and trap the evil spirit in it. The patient will be cured of the illness after the expulsion of *Muni* from his body.

Then the *Vichakkaran* will take magical threads, strands and yarns and tie the *Muni* firmly with them. Then he will be beaten thoroughly by a whip of fire. Afterwards, he will be immersed in deep sea. Then a screen made of fire will be erected in front of the sea to prevent his return from there. The screen of fire will be as high as the sky. All these things are carried out by the power of magic and they are not visible to the ordinary mortals.

c. '*Kattuchavar*' and Disease

Kattuchavar is one of the earth gods residing in the dense forest. He is a deity worshipped by the Muthuvans and is also called *Muthuvan Chavar*. There is another earth god known as *Uralichavar* residing in the thick of forests. He is an earth god propitiated by the *Uralies;* another tribal community of the area.

Both these benevolent gods may turn into malevolent ones occasionally. Diseases and other calamities can be caused due to their anger. A *Vichakkaran* can find out this matter by divination. He will prepare two pairs of iron rings. Two rings will be slightly smaller than the others. These rings are made to offer to the earth gods. Then the *Vichakkaran* will take these rings and go to the interior area of forest where no human habitation exists. After reaching there, the *Vichakkaran* will pluck two leaves and pack the iron rings in them as two packets. One small ring and a big one will be kept in one packet. Then the *Vichakkaran* will stand upright facing the eastern side, holding the ring packets in his right hand. In this posture, he will pray to the *Kattuchavar* and *Uralichavar* to heal the patient. He will also beg them to pardon the sins of the patient. After the prayer, the shaman will make two holes in the ground with a long stick and bury the packets separately, in the soil. After performing this ritual the patient will be healed from his disease.

d. Ancestral Spirits and Disease

The anger of ancestral spirits is one of the reasons for the occurrence of diseases. After the death of parents, their children have to fulfil the customary post-funeral ceremonies and other periodical offerings to appease them. If somebody failed to carry out this obligation, the ancestral spirits will get angry. They will retaliate for this omission, by sending diseases and other calamities to their relatives.

Through divination, a *Vichakkaran* can find out, whether the dead ancestors are angry. If so, a special ritual must be performed to appease their anger. This ritual is known as *Kumbidal.* A person who wants to perform this ritual will live in a separate house for one day. He will get up early the next morning, and after taking bath, go to the interior forest. When he reaches a place which is clean and tidy, he will stand on his knees facing the southern direction, and touch his forehead on the ground three times. Through imagination, he will then touch the feet of his dead ancestors and beg pardon for all his sins. Then he will pray to the dead ancestors, to heal his illness and protect him and all other members of his home from all calamities. The anger of dead ancestors will subside after performing this ritual, and the disease also will be healed within one or two days.

e. Evil Eye and Disease

The lustful gaze of a man or woman on the opposite sex can result in minor illnesses. The disease will develop on a person's face when he or she comes under the influence of the evil eye. Dry itches will appear on the cheek, lips and by the side of the nose. They will develop into a sore in the absence of proper treatment.

Some herbal remedies are efficacious in curing this disease. The tender leaves of a plant known as *Pichakam* (Jasminam grandiflorum) have to be collected and ground well to make it a paste. Afterwards this paste has to be mixed with the saliva of a woman living in the neighbourhood and applied over the sore. After two hours the medicine can be washed away using cold water. Application of the medicine has to be continued for two days to effect complete cure.

The saliva is mixed with the herbal paste to neutralize the evil influence of the gaze. When the sore develops on the face of a woman, the saliva of a man has to be used and vice versa. The saliva of the members of the patient's household is not suitable.

If the medicine fails to cure the sore after two days, then it has to be rubbed with the long hair of a woman living in the neighbourhood. Rubbing the sore with the beauty spot or the eyeliner taken from the face of a woman is yet another method of treatment.

f. Breach of Taboo and Disease

The Mannans observe some taboos in their community life. Most of them have originated from the belief in the supernatural forces. So their violation invites the wrath of supernaturals and they will send diseases and other calamities to the human beings, to teach them a lesson. Therefore the Mannans are very particular in following these taboos. If somebody happened to violate them, he will make the necessary offerings in the temple and observe other rituals for the expiation of his sins. Some of the important taboos of the Mannans are the following:

1. Eating the meat of cow, buffalo and elephant is a taboo. Cow is considered the mother of man, as it gives milk. Only her milk can be used. Eating the meat of a cow is an unpardonable sin.

2. Wearing shoes or sandals made of leather, as leather is prepared from the skin of cow or buffalo.

3. Sleeping on a cot is a disgraceful act towards earth goddess. One should lie on the floor as a child sleeps on his mother's lap.

4. For men, going to the menstrual hut is a taboo. Such a man will be considered polluted.

5. Walking over the rope of a cow, by which it is tied to a tree or a stump is a disrespectful act towards the cow goddess.

6. Walking over a place where somebody has urinated or defecated is a taboo and will impart pollution to a person.

7. Bringing the flesh of a game from which blood is dripping, into an agricultural field is a taboo. Such an act will provoke the anger of earth gods.

8. Entry of a menstruating woman into a crop field is a taboo. Her presence will be harmful to the crops.

g. The Magical Poison and Disease

Magical poison or *Kaivisham* is a method employed by a sorcerer to harm another person. This mysterious poison can be given to a person, either through food, drinks or by magical means, without being noticed by him. Some sticky substances like pieces of finger nail, chaff, hair, small ants, etc., will be included in the magical poison. These things will stick on the inner wall of the human intestine. The vicious magical power of a sorcerer can stay on the body of a person, through these articles and he can also influence the mind of the patient through them. Such a person will lose the vigour of the body and mind, and often become a drunkard. He will also suffer from belly pain and fatigue.

The diseases as a result of the effect of magical poison cannot be cured easily, as the poison is sticky in nature. The poison will persist there for indefinite time and cause various troubles to the patient. Only some temporary relief can be obtained through medical treatment. For achieving a permanent and complete cure, the substances stuck on to the intestinal wall must be removed, and thrown out of the body. Only some magical means will help to achieve this end.

h. Gods and Disease

The Mannans believe that for maintaining general health and well being, the goodwill of gods is quite essential. So they propitiate them and also make periodical offerings, to maintain their pleasure. Gods are generally benevolent in nature. But they will turn into malevolent ones when people provoke them through evil deeds. The angry gods will send diseases and other calamities to people to punish them. *Mariyamma* is one of the chief goddesses who get angry easily. Besides smallpox, chickenpox and measles, she will cause skin diseases, fever and belly pain. Some of the jungle gods like *Nayanachy* and *Kulachavar* can cause accidents to people, while they roam in the wild forest.

People used to make vows that certain offering shall be made to a particular god for getting a favour from him. If a person fails to fulfil that vow after receiving the favour, the god will get angry and will send various diseases to him as a punishment.

i. Curse and Illness

The Mannans believe that the curse of parents and other elders has some destructive power and can effect much harm to the children. The curse can bring about diseases, crop failures and accidents. So the children are very careful, to avoid the causes which will provoke the parents, and thus avoid receiving any curse from them.

j. Aanakali And Pulikali

Certain beliefs known as *Aanakali* and *Pulikali* exist among the Mannans. *Aanakali* means wrath of the elephant and *Pulikali* means wrath of the tiger or leopard. After an elephant or leopard had killed an individual in the forest, others will be very much afraid, to pass through that part of the forest. They will have fear about the elephant or leopard and imagine that it will again return and kill more people. So they cannot roam in the forest freely, when this fright is lingering in their mind.

An *Aanavathy* and a *Pulivathy* can neutralize this fright with the help of some magical rituals. Besides the rituals to quell fright about the elephant and leopard, they will also perform some ceremonies to appease the restless soul of the person who was killed by the elephant or leopard. After neutralizing the fright, the people can roam in the forest without any fear in their mind.

MAGIC AS MEDICINE

The Mannans have a well developed ethnomedical system as a part of their traditional culture. As their abode was the dense forests, they had invented their medicines from the plants available there. Some animal and mineral matter also was used as the ingredients of their medicine. So, their system of medicine was evolved from nature and was quite suitable for checking the diseases that occurred to them. The religious beliefs and myths played a major role in influencing their ethnomedical practices. Therefore shamanism became an integral part of ethnomedicine and it played the leading role over material herbal medicine. Thus shamanism and herbal remedies can be considered as the two basic components of ethnomedical system.

There is a belief existing among the Mannans, that the medicine was first invented by the *Vathykal* (pl.). In the remote past, there was only magic, by which the *Vathykal* manipulated the supernatural powers and cured their patients. With the passing of time they noticed that all the diseases are not healed, merely by chanting the spells. So they started giving material medicine also to the patients, besides performing the magical rituals. However, they gave more emphasis to the spells and rituals, while the material medicine had only a supplementary role.

The material medicine might have been first invented through a trial and error method. The primitive man might have noticed that even carnivorous animals were eating some herbs occasionally. Then he might have invented the curative value of some plants by a careful observation of the habits and experiences of these animals.

When somebody is sick in a household, other members of the house will pray to the gods and ancestral spirits to save the patient from the disease and restore his health. Normally, the severity of the illness will diminish after this prayer. If it continues it will then be construed, that the patient has done something which invoked the anger of god. Then he will be taken to a *Vichakkaran* and he will diagnose the disease through some divination techniques known as *Kodanki.* Through divination he will find out the cause of the illness and its remedy.

Usually, the Mannans will not immediately go for medicine when affected by a disease. If the illness is not serious, they will take rest in their homes and sit in the sun for a long time. If the illness is not healed after two or three days, they will go for some medical help. The elders in the household will give him some home remedies in the meantime.

DIVINATION TECHNIQUES

At the time of divination, the *Vichakkaran* presents the problem of disease, before the supernaturals, seeks their opinion about its cause and remedy. The supernatural beings are thus getting involved in the treatment procedure through the deliberate action of the *Vichakkaran.* In a way, the supernaturals are invited by the *Vichakkaran* to tackle the problem of illness. With their help he is making amends for his limitations.

Divination is the first phase in the treatment of a patient. This phase will reveal a clear picture of the patient and the cause of his present trouble to the *Vichakkaran*. This clear idea about the patient and his problems, will help the *Vichakkaran* to decide, what kind of remedy will be appropriate to heal his illness.

KODANKI

The Mannans have a special divination technique known as, *Kodanki*, to find out the cause of a disease and its probable remedy. Why the patient is affected by this disease; which god is angry with the patient; whether the disease is due to sorcery and if so, who is the sorcerer, etc., are problems that could be solved through *Kodanki*.

A footstool will be used as the divination board. Paddy grains also are used in the divination process. First the *Vichakkaran* will sit on the floor and keep the divination board in his front. Then he will take one or two pinches of paddy grains and keep them in one corner of the divination board. After this, the diviner will close his eyes and meditate for a while. He will call the god *Kadal Mulluran* whose abode is the sea in the west. He is the creator of paddy grains. Then all other local jungle gods and ancestral spirits will be invoked. All of them will help the *Vichakkaran* to obtain the correct result.

He will now start spreading the paddy grains on the divination board in a particular manner. He will take two grains each at a time and arrange them in three rows, without being touched by each other. He will remove two grains each, till all the grains are finished. In the end if only one grain is left, then it will be concluded that there is no fault with the patient. If two grains are left, then it is assumed that there is something wrong with the patient and that god is angry with him. Then all the paddy grains will be gathered together and the same process will be repeated to know what the remedy is, or what offering has to be made to god for the expiation of his sins. Other causes of disease like sorcery, intrusion of an evil spirit, etc. can be found out by employing the same technique with the paddy grains.

POLIVA

The divination process will show which god is angry and what offering has to be made to appease his anger. Then adequate offerings will be made in the temple. Sometimes, the offerings will be kept in the house for a certain period, often for one year. This is known as *Poliva.*

If a dhothi (cloth) is to be offered, a new dhothi will be purchased from the market, packed in green leaves, and then hung on the roof. Coins of money also will be kept like this, in the roof. This *Poliva* will be offered in the temple after one year or so. They believe that keeping of *Poliva* in a house will invoke the blessings of god.

PEYATTAM

This is a divination ritual employed, when the *Kodanki* method fails to give results. Some of the powerful evil spirits can interfere in the working of the divination method using the paddy grains, and withhold the results. In such situations the powerful *Vathykal* will adopt the *Peyattam* method of divination.

A Vathi will not have any special attachment towards a particular god or jungle spirit. At the time of divination, he will call all the gods, jungle spirits and ancestral deities. Besides them, there is another group of super natural entities known as *Kannikal* (Pl) who are very helpful to a shaman in both divination and treatment of disease.

At the time of divination, the shaman will first invoke the gods, ancestral spirits and jungle deities. The *Kannikal* who are a little inferior to the gods, will be invoked only later. They are invited by singing a particular song, asking their help. The *Vathy* will play a fiddle when he sings to invoke the *Kannikal.* There will be a special lustre when the *Kannikal* arrive and only the *Vathy* can see them. The *Vathy* will be possessed by them at the end of the song and will *be* in a trance state for some time. In that mental ecstasy, he will jump to the courtyard and dance in a wild fashion. His steps will be very swift, with face directed towards the sky. This magical dance is known as *Peyattam.* In that ecstasy, the *Vathy* will utter a few words in a strange tone. It is believed that this is not his original voice, but that the *Kannikal* are speaking through him. Through these words, they will announce the reason behind the occurrence of the disease and what offerings and sacrifices are to be made for its remedy.

The *Vathy* will return to his normal state of mind after the revelation of the *Kannikal* and conclude his ecstatic dance. Then he will perform the healing rituals depending upon the disclosures made by the *Kannikal*, about the cause and remedy of the illness. He will also order the relatives of the patient to act according to the directions of the *Kannikal*.

USE OF MEDICINE IN MAGIC

Besides the knowledge in magic, most of the *Vichakkaranmar*, have expertise in the curative properties of a number of medicinal plants. They make use of the expertise of both branches in their treatment. When a patient is brought to him, occasionally he may give some material medicine to him, before commencing the divination and healing rituals. He will chant various spells while giving this medicine to the patient and is often considered as a part of magic.

To cite an example, a patient suffering from belly pain may be given a simple medicine first. For preparing this medicine, the *Vichakkaran* will take a small quantity of water in a tumbler and then pour a few drops of coconut oil over it. Then he will take one burning charcoal and put it in the glass. Soon white fumes will emerge as the oil gets ignited. Then he will close the tumbler with his palm, for preventing the fumes from going out. When the fume ceases, the charcoal will be taken out, and the solution will be stirred thoroughly. Then it will be given to the patient to drink. While preparing the solution, and giving it to the patient, the *Vichakkaran* will chant a number of spells, to divert the attention of the patient.

Actually the solution itself is a medicine, and the *Vichakkaranmar* confess that the spells have nothing to do with it. However, for a patient having deep faith in the efficacy of magic, the spells and rituals have a psychological impact on him and in a way increase the efficacy of medicine. The patient will be more confident, by watching that necessary spells are being chanted to relieve his pain. Actually, the material medicine is playing the major role for his relief, without being recognized by him.

Here, the *Vichakkaran* is acting in two ways. Firstly he gives a simple medicine to his patient which can give him some immediate symptomatic relief. Secondly, through chanting spells he drives away the mental agony of the patient and brings confidence in him by making him realize that something is being done to relieve his pain. However, the spells and rituals will get emphasis over the medicine that the patient is taking. After this preliminary step, which will normally give an initial relief to the patient, further more complicated magical rituals will be performed by the shaman, which will give total relief to him.

HEALING RITUALS

The healing rituals constitute an integral component of the treatment procedure of a Mannan *Vichakkaran*. The rituals are usually performed after the phase of divination. They function as devices to ward off the evil forces creating trouble in the patient, and also restore the goodwill of gods. As many of the diseases originate due to the anger of god or ancestral spirits, the patient will be outside of the protective umbrella of the supernaturals at that time. Through the rituals the *Vichakkaran* will repair the broken relationship between the supernaturals and the patient and bring him under their protective cover once again. He will also order the patient to make appropriate offerings to god as a token of his repentance. Thus, through the ritualistic medium, the *Vichakkaran* is acting as a mediator between god and the patient.

In the case of the intrusion of an evil spirit, the shaman will act as the guardian of the patient's body and mind. Through divination, he will find out the wicked forces and by means of his powerful magical rituals, he will attack them. He will invoke the benevolent deities for assisting him in this operation. After warding off the evil spirits, the *Vichakkaran* will perform some rituals to prevent their return.

The healing rituals are quite relevant for the patient also. Even though he may not be in a position to understand the various manipulations of the *Vichakkaran*, he will surely get an impression that the shaman is really trying hard to eradicate the illness with the assistance of supernatural forces. This favourable mental disposition will help him to develop an anticipatory hope for a cure. Some of the important healing rituals of the Mannans are given below.

1. Breach of taboo and disease

Munthiya-dikkuka

When a standing crop attains maturity, the Mannans used to erect a magical fence around the field with the help of *Vathykal*. This invisible fence is constructed in order to prevent the attack of wild animals and sorcerers of other communities. If a sorcerer tries to trespass on the field he will be injured by the weapons attached to the fence. The men of the hamlet and the women who are not in their mensus period can enter the field. It will be fatal for a menstruating woman to enter such a crop field. Her presence will be harmful for the crop also. If such a woman happened to enter a field, she will be wounded by the weapons fixed on the magical fence and will die from profused bleeding.

A woman hurt by the magical fence and bleeding profusely through the vagina, will be taken to the *Vathy* who has originally constructed this magical fence. Only he can save this woman through some magical techniques. The *Vathy* will make the woman sit on the ground with her face, legs and hands directed towards the west. Then he will take a white cloth without any border and beat her twelve times with it from the head to the feet. He will chant a number of spells while beating the woman. The magical weapons like knives, swords, chisels, spears etc. will be removed by thorough beating. This ritual is known as *Munthiyadikkuka* in the Mannan dialect. The bleeding will cease after the removal of the weapons from the woman's body.

2. Snake Poison and Magic

Magic is very effective in combating snake poison. There are also so many herbal remedies to heal snake poison. The herbalist prepares his medicine, depending upon the kind of snake which bit the patient. If a person cannot identify the snake which bit him, the herbalist *(Vaidyan)* will not be able to treat that patient. Then he will be taken to a *Vichakkaran*.

The *Vichakkaran* will wash the wound with fresh water and squeeze out the blood from the mouth of the wound. Then the wound will be wiped with a dry cloth. With his forefinger he will then draw a line above the wound, using lime. He will chant spells while drawing the line. Then a herbal medicine prepared as a paste, will be applied over the top of the patient's head. The line of lime is drawn in order to prevent the venom from spreading in the blood. If the venom comes up over that line, a second and then a third line will be drawn a little above the first one. Usually the venom will not come above the third line.

If the, venom cannot be controlled at the region of the third line, the case will be hopeless and shaman will give up that patient. It is quite interesting that no medicine is consumed inside the body.

3. Measles, Chickenpox And Smallpox

These diseases constitute a special category, as all of them are supposed to be caused by the wrath of goddess *Mariyamma.* Therefore no material medicine is efficacious to check them. If somebody dares to consume medicine, it will aggravate the anger of the goddess and the patient's condition will become worse.

When a person is affected by this disease, he will be given a separate room or sometimes all other members may go to another house in the neighbourhood. The patient will be given special plates for taking food, and there are also some restrictions in the diet. Usually he will be given only gruel and side dish prepared without using any spice, salt or oil. During those days they will not fry anything in oil. They believe that the goddess *Mariyamma* does not like the smell of oil and spice and using these items will aggravate her anger.

After seven days of secluded life, the patient will be brought to the courtyard of his house and made to stand there. The *Vichakkaran* of that hamlet and other household members will gather around him. The *Vichakkaran* will place a new, unused broom on the head of the patient. Sometimes, a small quantity of turmeric paste also will be placed along with the new broom. Then seven pots of fresh water will be poured over his head, one after another. The *Vichakkaran* will utter some prayers to appease *Mariyamma* while pouring the water. After this ritual, he will take the broom from the patients head and pat all over his body with it. Spells will be chanted in loud voice, while doing this ritual, which is intended to ward off the goddess *Mariyamma* from the patient's body. She does not like a broom and when touched by a broom, she will soon vacate that place.

This is the only ritual performed to eradicate the disease and appease the goddess. In majority of the cases, the disease will be cured after conducting this ritual. If it is not healed after the ritual, then nothing more can be done to get rid of it. The patient may either die or may get well after a period of time.

4. Magical Poison And Its Cure

The magical poison send by a sorcerer can cause numerous troubles in a person. As stated earlier it can bring a number of body ailments like belly pain, dysentery, ulcer, headache and chronic fatigue. The poison can also affect the mind and cause mental derangement. So he will become lazy and a drunkard in due course of time.

The diseases originating from magical poison can be cured completely by eradicating the poisonous materials deposited in the intestine. A combined use of both medicine and magic will be essential for successfully carrying out this operation. The assistance of supernaturals also will be needed to carry out this programme. The help of a jungle god known as *Maivar* and also the service of *Kannikal* will be specially sought to undertake the cleaning process inside the body of the patient.

This kind of magical treatment is usually employed only to heal such type of diseases which could not be checked even after taking medicines for a prolonged period. Through divination, a *Vathy* can find out the presence of magical poison inside the body of the patient.

The ceremony for warding off the magical poison will be conducted in the patient's house. A special ground will be prepared in the centre of the courtyard for carrying out the ritual. The boundaries of this square shaped ground will be demarcated using some indigenous colours like turmeric powder, charcoal powder or rice flour. A kindled oil lamp will be placed in the centre of the ground. The atmosphere will be filled with the smoke and sweet smell of burning incences. The *Vathy* will bring holy water, holy ash and a cane and place them in one corner of the ground. Flowers of Chrysanthus can be seen floating over the holy water.

Then the patient will be brought to this special ground and made to sit in one corner. He has to take bath and wear new clothes before arriving there. The *Vathy* will come and sit in the opposite corner of the ground. Before starting the ritual proper, the *Vathy* will take some holy ash and smear it on the forehead of the patient. He will also sprinkle some holy water over the patient and give him a little of it to drink.

Then the *Vathy* will sit on the ground and start chanting a number of spells. Through these spells he will invoke the god *Maivar*, local jungle gods, ancestral spirits and the seven *Kannikal*. The *Vathy* will assign specific duty to each of the *Kannikal* who are acting as his helpers. With their arrival the *Vathy* will reach a trance state. The *Kannikal* being supernatural entities could attain any shape or form and enter anywhere they want.

After being possessed by the *Kannikal*, the *Vathy* will take the cane (Calamus rotang) in his hand. This cane will have three joints and is specially prepared for magical purposes. The *Vathy* himself will cut this from the dense forest and give it power through some magical means.

By holding this cane, the *Vathy* will order one *Kanny* to go inside the patient's body. She will enter the intestine of the patient and pull off all the poisonous substances stuck on its wall.

The *Vathy* will wait for sometime, after sending the *Kanny* into the body of the patient. Then he will put one end of his cane into the mouth of the patient. The other end will be kept in his mouth and he will suck forcibly through it. Even though the cane is not hollow, the poisonous materials inside the patient's intestine are supposed to rise upwards and enter the mouth of the shaman, by the power of the magic. Then the *Vathy* will spit them out. Usually he will tie a cloth firmly around his throat, to prevent the poisonous materials from accidentally entering his body and hurting him. The poison will be coming out very speedily and the *Vathy* must be very careful to spit it out, just as it enters his mouth. Actually the *Kanny* inside the intestine of the patient is supposed to be pushing the poison upwards, when the *Vathy* sucks through the cane from outside. The poisonous materials taken out from a patient include spiders, cockroaches, beetles, nail clippings, hair, small stones, etc.

After clearing the poison from the intestine, the *Kanny* will clean the inside of the patient. Blood may come out while she forcibly pluck the poisonous things stuck on the intestinal wall. She will wash these wounds using the holy water in the stomach. For this cleaning purpose, the shaman gives some holy water to the patient to drink at the initial stage of the warding off ceremony. After washing the wounds, she will wipe away the blood and all other unwanted materials, using her divine cloth brought from the spirit-world. She will return to the shaman after the cleaning is over. So the patient will be very pure, healthy and free from all evil after the completion of this magical ceremony. His disease also will be healed permanently as the magical poison is completely removed from the body.

After this ceremony, the *Vathy* will invoke some benevolent deities and put the patient under their protection. A male will be put under a god and a female under a goddess. So they will take care of the patients in future and resist every attack directed towards them by evil spirits or sorcerers.

TALISMAN

The Mannan shamans know the technique of preparing talisman and they believe in its protective power. It is known as *Virappu* in their dialect. A talisman will protect a person who wears it from the attack of evil spirits, fright and certain diseases. So it can be considered as a prophylactic measure.

For preparing a talisman, a *Vichakkaran* will first take a paddy grain and chant some spells to impart magical power to it. Then it will be packed in a small piece of paper and tied firmly using a thread. It will then be enclosed in a small tube made of either silver or iron. Afterwards, the shaman will tie this talisman either on the waist or on the neck of a person, using a black thread. Each talisman will be powerful for a certain period only. After that specific time the magical power of talisman will return to the *Vichakkaran*. Then a new talisman is to be prepared, if the person needs it.

A person who wears a talisman has to follow some moral codes and lead a good life for enjoying its benefits. The shaman will inform these matters to the person while giving him the talisman. If the man violates these rules, the magical power of the talisman will return to the *Vichakkaran*. He has also the power and authority to withdraw the power of a talisman if the behaviour of its wearer is not proper.

GOD-THE SCAPEGOAT

The *Vathykal* as well as *Vichakkaranmar* are such a breed of professionals who will not accept failure while combating with diseases and evil spirits. Fellow members of the community respect them for their knowledge in shamanism, medicinal plants and the ability to contain various diseases. For preserving this social prestige, they will take up any case of illness brought to them.

Really, the shamans know that they will not be able to cure all kinds of diseases. But they do not want to tell this truth openly to their clients. So when they fail in checking a certain disease, they will simply tell the patient or his relatives that the wrath of god prevents the success of their treatment. Through their divination methods, they will find that the patient had committed a number of misdeeds and consequently evoked the anger of god. Therefore the shamans will advise their patients to make some offerings in certain temples to appease the wrath of god, and then return to them for continuing the treatment.

The shamans will thrust the idea upon the patients that their healing rituals and medicine will be effective only after neutralizing the anger of gods. After a few days, the disease may subside automatically without the help of either medicine or magic. Then the healers will claim that the disease is cured by the effect of their medicine and magic and also as a reward for the offerings that are being made to gods, following their advice. With these kind of justifications, they will successfully conceal the failure of their treatment and maintain the faith of their clients.

Actually the shamans know, that it is due to the inefficacy of their treatment that the disease could not be controlled. They will lose their social prestige and power if they tell this fact openly to their clients. To avoid this unpleasant situation, the shamans accuse the gods for their failure. They are making gods responsible for all the trouble of their patients. Thus they succeed in maintaining their reputation as healers.

However, the real loser in this situation is the poor patient. He is not in a position to recognize the inability of the shamans and he only thinks that god is against him.

DEARTH OF SHAMANS

The *Vathy* plays an important role in the traditional life of the Mannans. He protects the tribe from all natural and supernatural calamities and ensures prosperity in the hamlet. After the death of a *Vathy* the protective magical fence around the hamlet will vanish and nobody will be there to prevent the wicked forces from entering the hamlet. So the members of the hamlet will soon try to find out a new *Vathy*, for continuing the mission of the old one.

In the present age, when a *Vathy* dies it is rather difficult, or even impossible to a certain extent, to find out a suitable candidate to fill this gap. The persons who possess the knowledge of magic or *Vicha* are very rare. The youngsters are not interested in learning *Vicha* from the old *Vathykal* or *Vichakkaranmar*. The elders opine that the youngsters are indifferent in learning *Vicha* and are giving little value for its utility in healing illnesses and averting calamities. The youngsters hold that magic is a mere superstition and only modern medicine can save them from diseases. Most of the old *Vathykal* are much distressed by these new developments and many of them believe that the practice of shamanism will come to an end with their death.

However, another facet of this problem also needs special mention. It is true that the present day youngsters are generally not interested in learning magic. But the attitude of the *Vathykal* also deters many of the interested persons from entering this profession. They put so many conditions and reservations in teaching them. In the case of most of the teachers, the most important spells are revealed only at their last moment, from their death bed. Often many of the important spells and techniques will be buried with them. So, with the passing of time, many of the efficacious spells and techniques are lost from traditional shamanism, and it affects the viability of the system.

ILLNESS AND THERAPEUTIC RECIPES

The names of common illnesses afflicting the people and the therapeutic recipes followed by the medicinemen of the Mannan community for the preparation of efficacious medicines to check them are given in the following pages. It is observed that some of the therapeutic recipes are common for both the Muthuvans and the Mannans. But they are not repeated in the list of therapeutic recipes given here.

1. *Thalavedana* (Headache)

a. Grind the leaves of *Aanachoriyanam* (Girardinia diversifolia) and apply this paste on the forehead.

b. Grind the root of *Kattupadavalam* (Trichosanthus cucumeriyana) and smear this paste on the forehead.

c. Mash the leaves of *Vettilakodi* (Piper betel) and the bulb of *Chuvannully* (Allium cepa) and extract the juice. Use this juice as an eye-drop.

d. Take some water in a shallow vessal and put some red hot pebbles into it. While steam emerge from the vessal, bent over it and receive it on the face. Cover the patient's head and the vessal with a blanket so that the steam would not escape.

2. *Nenchuvedana* (Chest pain)

a. Prepare a decoction by boiling the tubers of *Naruneendi* (Hemidesmus indicus) and *Chathavely* (Asparagus recemosus) in water and drink.

b. Prepare a decoction by boiling the roots of *Kurumthotti* (Sida rhombifolia) in water and drink.

c. Grind the leaves of *Nilappana* (Curculigo orchioides) with a little oil extracted from the seeds of *Veppu* (Azadirachta indica) and smear this paste on the chest.

3. *Murivu* (Wound)

a. Prepare a paste by grinding together the root of *Idampiri Valampiri* (Helicteres isora), the leaves of *Venapacha* (Blumea lacera), little soot, lime and a few crystals of common salt (NaCl) and apply on the wound.

b. Apply the sap, obtained by cutting the branches of Maruthu (Terminalia paniculata) or *Vatta* (Macaranga peltata), on the wound.

c. Apply the white powder found on the mid-rib of *coconut leaf (Cocos* mucifera) on the wound.

d. Grind the leaves of *Appa* (Ageratum conyzoides) and apply this paste on the wound.

e. Grind the tender shoots of *Edana* (Olea dioica) with a piece of the rhizome of *Manjal (Curcuma longa)* and apply this paste on the wound.

4. *Theeppollal* (Burn)

a. Grind the leaves of *Kattukachil* (Dioscorea bulbifera) and mix this paste with honey and soot obtained by burning hair and old cloth. Apply this mixture over the affected part.

b. Extract the oil of *Mathy* (a sea-fish) and apply over the affected part.

5. *Pani* (Fever)

a. Boil the leaves and flowers of *Thumba* (Leucas zeylanica) in water and take bath in this medicated water.

b. Boil *Veluthully* (Allium sativum) and *Vattal Mulaku* (red chilly) in the oil extracted from *Veppu (Azadirachta indica)* and massage the head and body with this medicated oil.

c. Prepare a decoction by boiling the rhizome of *Inchy (Zingiber officianel)*, seeds of *Pepper* (Piper nigrum) and leaves of *Thulasi* (Ocimum sanctum) and drink.

d. Boil a crab in water and eat it and drink that water.

e. Mash the tender stem of *Amruthu* (Tenospora cordifolia) and extract the juice. Mix the juice with honey and drink.

6. *Chuma* (Cough)

a. Prepare a decoction by boiling *Ully* (Allium cepa), *Inchy* (Zingiber officianel), pepper (Piper nigrum) and a crab in water; mix it with honey and drink.

b. Grind the fruits of *Theppoly* (Piper longum) with a little rock salt and take this paste.

7. *Nilamkarichuma* (Whooping cough)

Prepare a decoction by boiling the fruits of *Nagamulla* (Opuntia dillenii) in water and drink.

8. *Kannilasukham* (Eye disease)

a. Use *Cheruthen* (honey of small bees) as an eye-drop.

b. Cut the tender stem of *Chooral* (Calamus rotang) and pour a few drops of the sap in the eye.

9. *Vayarilakkam* (Dysentery)

a. Mash the bark of *Njaval* (Syzigium cumini), *Punna* (Calophyllum enophyllum) and *Pezhu* (Careya arborea) and drink the juice.

b. Grind the tender leaves of *Pera* (Psidium guava) and mix this paste with water and drink.

c. Mash the bark and root of *Analivegam* (Alstonia venenata) and extract the juice and drink.

d. Crush the shoot and tender stem of *Chandanavayambu* (UI) and drink the juice.

e. Prepare a decoction by boiling the leaves of *Poovamkurunnila* (Vernonia cineria) in water and drink.

f. Prepare hot tea and add lemon juice in it and drink.

g. Grind the leaves of *Vetta* (Piper betel) with common salt (NaCl) and fruits of *Kanthari* (Capsicum sp) and take this paste.

10. *Vayarukadi* (Diarrhoea with defecation of blood)

a. Grind the leaves of *Paval* (Momordica charantia) and drink the juice.

b. Grind the seeds of *Mathalam* (Punica granatum) and mix with the milk of goat and drink.

c. Dry the penis of a *Mlavu* (an elk) and crush it into a powder and take.

11. *Vayaruvedana* (Belly pain)

a. Grind the *Nilappala* (Euphorbia hirta) in toto and dilute with water and drink.

b. Mash the bark of *Unnam* (Grewia tilifolia) and drink the infusion.

c. Mash the *Kurumthotti* (Sida acuta) in toto and drink the infusion.

d. Grind together the tender fruit of *Chora* (*UI*), the rhizome of *Vellakuva* (Curcuma augustifolia) and the rhizome of *Kasturimanjal* (Curcuma aromatica) and dilute with water and drink.

e. Grind the rhizome of *Vayambu* (Acorus calamus) and take this paste. This paste can be smeared on the belly also.

f. Mix a few drops of the fat of bear in hot water and drink in the morning, before taking any food.

12. *Chory* (Scabies)

a. Grind the leaves, roots and seeds of *Nagamulla* (Rhinacanthus nasutus) and apply this paste on the affected part of the body.

b. Extract the oil from the seeds of *Elam* (Elettaria cardamomum) and apply on the scabies.

c. Grind the bark and roots of *Idampiri Valampiri* (Helicteres isora) and apply the paste on the affected portion of the body.

d. Grind the leaves and roots of *Kattupuli* (*UI*) and dilute with water and drink.

e. Extract the oil from the seeds of *Nanku* (Gnidia glauca) and apply on the scabies.

13. *Puzhukadi* (Ring-worm)

a. Grind a piece of *Sandalwood stem* (Santalum album) and apply this paste on the affected part of the body.

14. *Krumikadi* (Pin-worm)

a. Grind together the seeds of *Elam* (Elattaria cardamomum) and the rhizome of *Vellakuva* (Curcuma augustifolia) and consume this paste.

b. Grind the rhizome of *Vayambu* (Acorus calamus), dilute with water and drink.

15. *Virashalyam* (Tapeworm and roundworm infestation)

a. Mash the leaves and rhizome of *Channakuva* (Costus speciosus), dilute it with water and extract the juice by filtering through a cloth and drink.

b. Grind the seeds of *Kappalam* (Carica papaya) and mix this paste with hot water and drink.

c. Grind the leaves of *Aryaveppu* (Melia azadirachta) into a paste and take.

16. *Vayu* (Gas trouble)

a. Cut a *Lemon fruit* (Citrus aurantifolia) into small pieces and boil in water. Mix this with the juice obtained by crushing the leaves of *Panikurka* (Coleus aromaticus), and drink.

b. Grind the wood of *Kanjiram* (Strychnos nux-vomica) and mix with water and drink.

17. *Schardy* (Vomiting)

a. Crush the tuber of *Kacholam* (Campferia galanga) and drink the juice.

b. Grind the roots of *Anachuvadi* (Elephantopus scaber) and take this paste.

c. Mash the roots of *Poopoathiri* (Stereospermum chelonoides) and drink the juice.

18. *Constipation*

a. Eat the ripe fruits of *Koovalam* (Aegle marmelos).

b. Keep a little quantity of *Uluva* seeds (Trigonella foenum) in water and drink that water in the next morning.

19. *Arshasu (Piles)*

a. Grind the stem and leaves of *Changalamparanta* (Cissus quadrangularis) to make it a paste and take it in the morning for ten days.

b. Grind the tender leaves of *Mavu* (Mangifera indica) and smear that paste in the rectum.

c. Mash *Karukappullu* (Cynodon dactylon) in toto and drink the juice.

20. *Pampukadi* (Snake bite)

a. Grind the bark of *Analivegam* (Alstonia venenata) into a paste and take.

b. Grind the ripe inflorescence of *Kanchavu* (Cannabis sativa) with the fruits of *Kanthari* (Capsicum sp) and take this paste. Smear this paste on the wound`also.

c. Grind together a piece of camphor, bark of *Murikku* (Erythrina indica) and the roots of *Kattamara* (Dolichos trilobus). Mix this paste with the urin of that person whom the snake bit and drink.

d. Mash the bark of *Kachapatta* (Pittosporum nepalensis) and drink the juice.

e. Grind the bark of *Inthu* (Cycas circinalis) and apply this paste on that portion of the body where the snake bit.

f. Grind the leaves and stem of *Nagavally* (UI) and apply this paste on the mouth of the wound.

21. *Pattikadi* (Dog bite)

a. Grind *Aanachuvady* (Elephantopus scaber) in toto and apply on the wound.

b. Grind together the leaves of *Veppu* (Azadirachta indica) and the rhizome of *Manjal* (Curcuma longa) and apply this paste on the wound.

c. Prepare a decoction by boiling the dry seeds of *Ummam* (Datura stramonium) and *Thazhuthama* (Borhavia diffusa) in toto in water and drink.

d. Grind the leaves of *Snehapullu* (UI) with lime and smear this paste on the mouth of the wound.

22. *Manjapitham* (Jaundice)

a. Prepare a decoction by boiling *Nilappana* (Curculigo orchioides) in toto in water and drink.

b. Mash the tuber of *Shatavari* (Asparagus recemosus) and drink the juice.

c. Crush the tuber of *Naruneendi* (Hemidesmus indicus) with the tender roots of *Coconut* (Cocos mucifera) and drink the juice.

d. Prepare a decoction by boiling the leaves and seeds of *Kattamara* (Dolichos trilobus) and the leaves of *Sankaracheera* (Amaranthus sp) in water and drink.

e. Grind the leaves of *Kizhanelly* (Phyllanthus niruri) with a little quantity of cumin seeds and dilute this paste with hot water and drink.

f. Prepare a decoction by boiling the roots of *Vetty* (Aporusa lindleyana) in water and drink.

23. *Apasmaram* (Epilepsy)

a. Mash the leaves and bark of *Kanjiram* (Strychnos nux-vomica) and prepare a decoction by boiling it in water and drink.

b. Crush the *Brahmi plant* (Bacopa monnieri) in toto and extract the juice and drink.

c. Crush the seeds of *Kara* (Elaeocarpus tuberculatus) and boil them in water to prepare a decoction and drink.

24. *Shwasammuttal (Asthma)*

a. Prepare a decoction by boiling the roots of *Nilappana* (Curculigo orchioides) in water and drink. Take a little jaggery while drinking the decoction.

b. Prepare a soup using the flesh of a crow and drink.

c. Prepare a decoction by boiling the root of *Kunni* (Abrus precatorius) in water and drink.

25. *Kushtam* (Leprosy)

a. Prepare a decoction by boiling the roots of *Thottavady* (Mimosa pudica) and the bark of *Vaka* (Albizia lebbeck) in water and drink.

b. Extract the oil from the seeds of *Odal* (Sarcostigma kleinii) and apply on the affected part of the body.

c. Crush the bark of *Vedivempu* (Toona ciliata) and apply the juice on the affected portion of the body.

26. *Neeru* (Oedima)

a. Grind the bark of *Kumpil* (Melina arboria) into a paste and apply on the body.

b. Roast the leaves of *Aavanakku* (Ricinus communis) and tie them firmly over the affected portion of the body with a cloth.

27. *Vatham* (Rheumatism)

a. Prepare a decoction by boiling the crushed leaves and unripe fruits of *Ambazham* (Spondias pinnata) in water and drink.

b. Extract the oil from the fruits of *Kattunarakam* (Atalantia malabarica) and apply externally on the body.

c. Mash the leaves of *Iringil* (Alangium salvifolium) and pack in a cloth and apply as a poultice.

d. Extract the oil from the seeds of *Karinjota* (Quassia indica) and massage the body with it.

e. Prepare a decoction by boiling the roots of *Kurumthotti* (Sida rhombifolia) in water and drink.

28. *Ulukku* (Sprain)

a. Grind together the root of *Idampiri Valampiri* (Helicteres isora) and a piece of the wood of *Chandanam* (Santalum album) and smear this paste on the affected portion of the body.

b. Grind the leaves of *Njarampuri* (*UI*) and apply this paste on the affected part of the body.

29. *Chathavu* (Bruise)

a. Mash a small *Kanthari plant* (Capsicum sp) in toto and mix the juice with the urine of the patient and drink.

b. Grind the tender shoots of *Muringa* (Moringa olifera) with common salt (NaCl) and cumin seeds and dilute with hot water and drink.

30. *Thondaveekam* (Tonsilitis)

a. Extract the juice of the *Muyalchevian plant* (Emilia sonchifolia) and boil with equal quantity of coconut oil and apply on the head. A paste obtained by grinding the leaves of *Muyalcheviyan* is applied over the throat.

31. *Vayilkuru* (Sore throat)

a. Extract the pulp from the fruits of *Vilarmaram* (Feronia limonia) and smear it on the boils in the mouth.

b. Extract the juice from the fruits of *Panachi* (Diospyros peregrina) and use it as a gargle.

c. Crush the fruits of *Anachunta* (Solanum stramonifolium) and extract the juice and drink.

32. *Chevi vedana* (Ear ache)

a. Mash the tender leaves of *Ambazham* (Spondias pinnata) and extract the juice and use it as an ear-drop.

b. Extract the juice of the flowers of *Mula* (Bambusa arundinacea) and use it as an ear-drop.

c. Mash the rhizome of *Inchy* (Zingiber officianel) and extract the juice. Use the warm juice as an ear-drop.

33. *Pallu vedana* (Tooth ache)

a. Grind the *Kodangal plant* (Centella asiatica) in toto and smear the paste on the gums and cheek.

b. Use regularly the leaves of *Kattujathikka* (Myristica malabarica) for cleaning the teeth.

c. Prepare a decoction by boiling the leaves and root of *Venkurumthotti* (Abutilon indicum) in water and use it as a mouth wash.

d. Grind the tooth of elephant and use this powder for cleaning the teeth.

34. *Raktham pokku (Bleeding of women)*

a. Grind *Kizhanelly* (Phyllanthus niruri) in toto and mix this paste with the water obtained while washing the rice and drink.

b. Prepare a decoction by boiling the crushed bark of *Ashokam* (Saraca indica) in water and drink.

35. *To check the problems at the time of delivery*

a. Mash the roots of *Kurumthotti* (Sida acuta) and boil in cow's milk to prepare a decoction. Allow the pregnant woman to drink this decoction.

b. Prepare a decoction by boiling the *Cherula* (Erva Ianata) in toto with the tuber of *Naruneendi* (Hemidesmus indicus), in water and drink.

36. *Contraceptive for women*

a. Crush the bark of *Kattumavu* (Mangifera sp) and drink the juice continuously for one week. Then that woman become infertile for one month. Repeat the medicine in every month if the couple want to avoid pregnancy for long periods.

37. *Moothram chudil* (Inflammation of the urethra)

a. Prepare a decoction by boiling the leaves and roots of *Karinkurinji* (Strobilanthus heynianus) in water and drink.

b. Crush the fruits of *Cheruviri* (Cordia dichotoma) and drink the juice.

c. Prepare a decoction by boiling the *Poovankurunthal* (Vernonia sineria) in toto in water and drink.

38. *Ushnam (Venereal diseases)*

a. Crush the dried seeds of *Kattuvazha* (Musa superba) and mix this powder with cow's milk and drink continuously for one month.

b. Prepare a decoction by boiling the leaves, bark and root of *Mayirmanikkam* (Sida spinosa) in water and drink.

c. Crush the leaves of *Kakkappoovu* (Torenia asiatica) and extract the juice and drink.

d. Prepare a decoction by boiling the *Kallurukki* (Pouzolzia zeylanica) in toto, in water and drink.

39. *Paruvu* (Abscess)

a. Grind the tender leaves of *Thakara* (Casia tora) and apply this paste on the abscess.

b. Grind the shoot of *Cheruthekku* (Clerodendrum seratum) and smear this paste on the abscess.

40. *For the increased proudction of Breast-Milk*

a. Cut the tuber of *Palmuthukku* (Ipomea paniculata) into small pieces and boil in cow's milk and drink.

b. Grind the tuber of *Muthanga* (Cyperus rotundes) and smear this paste on the breast.

41. *Daham* (Excessive Thirst)

a. Extract the juice from the ripe and fresh fruits of *Athi* (Ficus racemosa) and mix with a little honey and drink.

42. *Valam Kadi* (Sores between the fingers of the leg)

a. Apply the sap of the *Erukku* (Calotropis gigantia) on the affected part.

ETHNOMEDICINE AND CHANGE

The system of ethnomedicine is now passing through a phase of transition. Availability of various medicinal plants has been facing a threat due to large-scale deforestation. The scarcity of medicinal plants is a great handicap in the treatment of certain diseases. Absence of some of the constituents decrease the efficacy of the medicinal combinations.

The changes that have occurred in the subsistence pattern of the Mannans also influence the ethnomedical system. The Mannans had no access to modern medicine when they were wandering in the forest as shifting cultivators. So, ethnomedicine was the only device to check diseases in those days. Modern medicine is now easily available to them after becoming settled agriculturalists and agricultural labourers.

Today ethnomedicine is facing great challenge from other systems of medicine like allopathy and ayurveda. As a part of the welfare programmes, the government has started a number of dispensaries, Primary Health Centres (PHC) and hospitals in the tribal areas. The easy availability of modern medicine attracted the Mannans, and after an initial period of hesitation and doubt, they have accepted its worth.

However, the old people of the community continue to support ethnomedicine. They opine that ethnomedicine is more effective, harmless and appropriate for the body, than modern medicine. They believe that, even though modern medicine can bring quick relief, it has so many other disadvantages. The harmful elements of modern medicine can remain in the body and effect new disease after a lapse of time.

Even though, a number of people are now utilizing modern medicine, one cannot write off the relevance of ethnomedicine. Still considerable number of people are approaching a *Vichakkaran* for healing their illnesses. While undergoing the treatment in a hospital, many people use to visit a *Vichakkaran* for getting his opinion about the cause of the disease. Many people believe that, the magic of *Vichakkaran* is very effective in healing diseases, especially when occurring due to the anger of gods, ancestral spirits and evil spirits. Along with modern medical treatment, they will make offerings in the temple as directed by the *Vichakkaranmar*. This is an example of peaceful co-existence of ethnomedicine along with modern medicine.

ETHNOMEDICINE OF THE MUTHUVANS AND THE MANNANS: SIMILARITIES AND DIFFERENCES

Ethnomedicine of the Muthuvans and the Mannans bears a number of similarities. Both communities show some resemblances regarding the structure and function of their medical system. Shamanism and herbal therapy are the two fundamental aspects of their ethnomedicine. Their concepts of etiology consist of both natural and supernatural causes, for the origin of diseases. There are a number of functionaries in both communities, who deal with the treatment of diseases. Their status and role are more or less same in both communities. They are not supposed to demand any reward for their service. In addition to shamanism, both Muthuvans and Mannans possess a well developed pharmacopoeia and a large number of therapeutic recipes as a part of their ethnomedicine. Some of the therapeutic recipes are common for both communities.

There are also some dissimilar features between the ethnomedicine of the Muthuvans and the Mannans. The Muthuvans believe that soul-loss is one reason for the occurrence of certain diseases. But the Mannans do not hold this belief. On the other hand, the Mannans believe that evil eye can cause some diseases. But the Muthuvans do not believe that evil eye is capable of bringing any disease.

The Muthuvan shamans are more powerful than their Mannan counterparts and they can even control certain supernatural entities. As mentioned earlier an *Aakaya Vathy* of the

Muthuvan Community can even control the goddess *Mariyamma* in such occasions when smallpox and/or measles attain the form of an epidemic. The Mannan shamans also accept that the magical techniques of the Muthuvan shamans are more powerful and efficacious than their own.

Animal sacrifice is a prominent feature of the healing rituals of the Muthuvans. They sacrifice hundreds of fowls and a considerable number of goats during their annual *Pongal* festival to fulfil the vows they have taken while afflicted by diseases. But, animal sacrifice is very rare among the Mannans in the present age. They have nearly abandoned this practice and do it only in great necessities.

The most important difference between the Muthuvans and the Mannans with respect to ethnomedicine is the way in which the two communities approach this system. Even though ethnomedicine is a part of their culture one can notice certain differences in the manner in which the two tribes treat their medical system. After the contact with the non-tribals and also after the introduction of modern medicine in the tribal areas the Mannans show much interest in exploiting the facilities of this new system of medicine, in addition to their ethnomedicine. For them ethnomedicine is having only a complementary role along with modern medicine. They do not show any preference for a particular system of medicine and avail the facilities of both systems according to the need of the circumstances. On the other hand the Muthuvans do not show any interest in accepting modern medicine and they still have ardent faith in ethnomedicine. As they are living isolated in the remote areas of forests, they have only limited experience with modern medicine. So their first preference is ethnomedicine and they are very reluctant to go to hospitals. They may go to hospital only when the disease is so serious and ethnomedicine could not cure it. Thus ethnomedicine has a good status in the Muthuvan community even today. On the other hand the Mannans living in the fringe areas of forests are giving more preference for modern medicine. The influence of outside agencies is one of the main reasons behind this differential behaviour between the Muthuvans and the Mannans. As mentioned earlier the Muthuvan community is very orthodox with a strong leadership. So it is very difficult for the new innovations to enter in such a conservative and tradition bound community. On the other hand the Mannan community is more acculturated and more receptive towards new innovations like modern medicine. The phenomenon of medical pluralism will be discussed in detail in the next chapter.

5

Health and Medical Pluralism

In recent years *'Health'* has been a much debated topic in both national as well as international arena. The *'Alma Ata Declaration'* of 1978, jointly proclaimed by the WHO and UNICEF is the major reason for this sudden interest of intellectuals, administrators, medical personnel and social workers of all countries on this topic. The catchy slogan of 'Health for all by 2000 A.D., provoked heated discussions and various forms of action in several countries. For the first time in history, the main emphasis is given to the importance and necessity of primary health care rather than modern curative medicine.

India also is a signatory of this well intentioned declaration made by the world bodies and a plan of action according to the guidelines of this programme has been drafted and implemented. In the spirit of the 'Alma Ata Declaration', the first priority has been given to National Health Policy which includes provision of health services to those residing in the tribal, hilly and backward areas as well as to endemic disease-affected populations and other vulnerable sections of the society (Statement on National Health Policy, 1982).

In the backdrop of this newly generated awareness, it will be interesting to look at the present health and sanitary conditions existing in the tribal communities. Even a casual observer can recognize that the tribals have to go a long way to attain the goals of good health and sanitary environment. Before formulating plans and the implementation of programmes, it is very necessary to evaluate the present situation and find out what are the factors hindering the attainment of health and sanitation, in the tribal communities.

The sanitary conditions and health of the Muthuvans and the Mannans are dealt with in the first part of the present chapter. In the latter part, an analysis of the impact of medical pluralism and its consequences in the health situation of the tribals is given. As there are little differences between the Muthuvans and the Mannans in this area, their common characteristics are analysed and presented jointly. To be sure, the conspicuous dissimilarities are mentioned separately for each tribe. The word 'tribal' is used while mentioning the common characteristics.

SANITARY CONDITIONS

The overall sanitary condition prevailing among the tribals is not satisfactory. There are many factors like poverty, ignorance, social customs, religious sanctions, age-old-habits, climatic conditions, etc., which play a role in the maintenance of a healthy sanitary atmosphere in the hamlets. As they are ignorant about the microorganisms and modes of infection they are least bothered about many of the unhygienic practices. They are not taking these things as anything harmful to their health and consider them as quite natural phenomena. Their sense of body cleanliness, eating habits, ablution practices, bathing habits etc. need modification for attaining a healthy standard.

HYGIENE OF THE HOUSE AND SURROUNDINGS

The tribals are careful to keep their house clean and tidy. Usually they will clean the floor of the house in the morning and evening with a broom made of the midribs of coconut leaflets. Since the floor of the house is plastered with either clay or a mixture of cow-dung and charcoal, the particles will always show a tendency to loosen themselves and stick on the body of the people. Therefore, it is very difficult to keep the floor clean and dust free.

Most of the houses have only one or two rooms including the kitchen. Because of the scarcity of space a lot of things like agricultural produces, tools, clothes, firewood, utensils, etc., can be seen dumped in the room. This messy arrangement gives plenty of opportunities for rats and some insects to thrive well among these things.

Usually the kitchen will be in the corner of the room and in some houses, there may be a separate room for the kitchen. The hearth will be always in the ground level and is usually made of three upright stones of about one to one and a half feet height. Utensils made of clay, aluminium and steel are generally used. They clean the utensils with clay, ash and the leaves of some herbs.

The Mannans usually collect the house refuse and throw it just outside the boundary of the courtyard. As the houses are arranged wide apart, this makes no sanitation problem. The houses of Muthuvans are arranged in clusters in close proximity with each other. So they collect the refuse and throw them away beyond the boundary of the hamlet. Usually the house refuse does not seem to make any problem for the environmental sanitation.

There is no provision for the removal of waste water and solid waste from the kitchen. After washing the utensils the women throw away the waste water in the backyard of the house. The continuous disposal of the waste water makes the courtyard filthy and causes the growth of algae. The food particles attract flies and insects which disseminate various types of diseases.

The tribals have a bad habit of spitting here and there. The Muthuvans even use to spit in the ashes of the hearth. The spittle attracts houseflies and can cause the spreading of disease if it contains any infectious microorganisms.

SOURCES OF DRINKING WATER

The tribals used to collect water from the natural sources like springs, rivers, ponds, brooks, etc. In a few hamlets the government have dug wells, but most of them get dried up in summer. The natural sources of water were very clean and hygienic in former times. Due to deforestation many of them no more exist. For the remaining ones, the chances of pollution are high because of the increase of population. Scarcity of drinking water is a big problem for the tribals during summer.

CAUSES OF WATER POLLUTION

There are some natural pollutants like algae and water-weeds which die and degenerate during summer. The humus accumulated in the bed of ponds and rivulets is another pollutant. They create problems during summer when the ponds and rivulets become shallow. The degenerating parts of water weeds and humus make the water filthy and unsuitable for human consumption.

Both the Muthuvans and Mannans empty their bowels in the open air and use the rivulets and ponds for cleaning purposes. This will pollute the water and cause a number of water borne diseases like diarrhoea etc. The same source of water is often used for ablution, bathing and drinking. This is an easy way for epidemics to spread from person to person through the medium of drinking water.

The Muthuvans are notorious for the evil practice of defecating in the rivulet itself. There may be small islands or big rock in the middle of small rivers and the Muthuvans use those places as their seats for easing themselves. They do it simply as a matter of convenience. During rain, all these faecal matter will be washed into the river. Karve says, "when people cannot afford to spend adequately even on food and clothing they do not just bother about environmental sanitation..... experience strengthens the view that sanitation is inextricably woven with the economic and social life of the people, and to the extent to which the latter improves, the sanitary consciousness of the people also correspondingly improves...... ' (quoted by Hasan, 1967:65).

PERSONAL HYGIENE

The tribals know the importance of personal hygiene and try to keep their body and clothes clean while moving around in the hamlet. But it is generally noticed that, while staying in the home, they use old and soiled clothes. As personal hygiene is the sum total of different habits and practices like defecation habits, bathing practices, ablution, cropping of hair, clothing, etc., each will be dealt with separately for getting a clear picture.

DEFECATION HABITS

Both the Muthuvans and the Mannans follow open air defecation. The adults get up around 5 a.m. and they go to the nearby forest for defecation. The Mannan women defecate in their agricultural fields or in the peripheral areas of forests. The Muthuvans never defecate in their crop fields. They consider their fields as divine places and pollution of such places will invoke the wrath of gods. However, the Muthuvans have the unhealthy practice of defecating in or near the forest rivulets which cause serious water pollution.

In a few hamlets, it is noticed that the Muthuvan men and male children defecate near the male dormitory. They are easing themselves just about 100 feet away from the dormitory. They empty their bowels in this place mainly during night, and very old men use it even during the day. As a number of people use the same spot, a pool of faeces develop there. This is an ideal breeding ground for flies, insects, microorganisms and numerous types of worms. The worst part of it is that after defecation they clean the parts simply by rubbing with the leaves or herbs in that bush. This may lead to fungal infection in the groin area.

The open air defecation also leads to soil pollution and consequently in the spreading of hook worm infection. As the tribals generally move around barefooted, the hook worm larvae can easily enter the body. The absence of sandals also can cause the infection of ring worms from the filthy mud pits.

The Muthuvan children sleeping in the male dormitory used to pass urine just near its entrance at night. After getting up in the night, they are very afraid to go to the boundary of the courtyard to pass urine, because they fear that evil spirits roam the earth at night. So they just come out of the hall and pass urine standing near the entrance. This will generate fowl smell and attract flies.

ABLUTION

After defecation they will go to the nearby water source and wash their parts. The Mannan men used to carry water in a pitcher if no water source is present near the spot of defecation. After ablution they are not bothered about the washing of hands.

CLEANING THE MOUTH

Both the Muthuvans and the Mannans clean

their mouth in the morning. After getting up in the morning they used to go to the nearby river or well for washing the mouth. Generally, they use a piece of charcoal or burnt husk of paddy for cleaning the teeth. They rub it on the teeth and gargle with water afterwards. Occasionally they use ripe leaves of mango tree (Mangifera indica) for cleaning the teeth. After the contact with the modern culture a few of the Mannans use tooth brush and paste for cleaning purpose. But their high cost do not permit them to use it widely. Some of them use the cheap tooth powder available in the market.

They use the midrib of the coconut leaflet as a tongue cleaner. They split the midribs to make its edges sharp. The children are not much particular in cleaning their tongue. While cleaning the teeth, they wash their face and eyes also.

CLEANLINESS OF THE HEAD

Both groups of tribes apply oil in their hair before taking bath. They use either coconut or gingelly oil for this purpose. They smear oil on the hands and legs also. Usually they comb their hair in the morning when they go out somewhere. The women usually comb their hair after completing the household chores of the morning. Sometimes a few women can be seen sitting around in the courtyard and picking lice from each other's heads. They spend this time by exchanging some local gossips.

Usually the condition of the hair of the little Muthuvan children is very poor. Often it can be seen tangled and soiled without any oil. The oil less hair often attains a copper or chestnut colour.

Sometimes, the Muthuvans grow the hair of their children to fulfil certain religious vows. When the children are affected by some diseases, the parents will make a vow that they will not cut the hair of that child for a certain period and afterwards visit that temple with the child. Children may grow their hair from six months to more than one year. Then the parents will take the child to that temple and shave its head. In some temples hair is considered as an offering to the deity. However, growing the hair of a child, without combing or applying oil is hazardous to its health. Such dirty hair will be infested with lices and may sometimes lead to skin diseases.

The tribals are not very particular in cutting the fingernails. The children often cut short the nails by biting. Their nails are often covered with dirt, which contains disease-causing microorganisms. They may enter the body along with the food and cause illness.

Women used to apply 'kanmashy' (collyrium) in the eyes to beautify themselves. They either purchase it from the market or use the carbon on the oil lamps (lampblack).

The men are not regular in shaving their face. Usually they shave their face once in a fortnight. Among the Mannans there are some persons who function as barbers for their fellowmen. They receive money for their service. Split pieces of reed were used for the shaving purpose in the past. Now they are using razor blades for the same. The Mannans crop their hair once in two months. Some of their shamans used to grow long hair. Traditionally, the Muthuvans grow long hair. But many of the young people now crop their hair after their initiation ceremony.

BATHING HABITS

The Mannans are much ahead of the Muthuvans in bathing practices. The men often take bath daily barring the old. The women usually bathe atleast twice in a week. Young women and children bathe daily.

The Muthuvans are not particular in taking bath daily. As they grow long hair, it will take a long time for them to dry it. So they take bath once in a week or so. The women are also following the same practice. However, children bathe more frequently than adults.

They take bath either in the rivers or in the ponds. In the past they were using the tender fruits of a tree, known as '*Pulinchy*' (Soapnut tree) as soap. Now they are using toilet soaps for washing their body. The bark of 'Incha' (Acacia caesia) plant is used as shampoo for cleaning the hair. Clothes are washed using washing soaps. In some places, Muthuvans have the habit of abandoning a washing soap after using it two or three times. They use cotton towels for wiping the water from the hair and body. They used to sit in the sun for a while, after taking bath.

All the members of a hamlet take bath on the annual festival day. For the Muthuvans it is the '*Thaipongal*' and for the Mannans it is the '*Makaravilakku*'. Without taking bath nobody can enter the premises of the temple of the hamlet on that day. They believe that the deities and ancestral spirits visit the hamlet on the festival day and everybody must be clean for receiving them.

The Mannan women have to take bath daily while they are staying in the menstrual hut. They believe that the body of a woman is polluted during the mensus period and she has to keep it clean always. Otherwise she may be possessed by some evil spirits during this unclean period. After confinement there is a ceremonial bath, usually on the third day. The woman bathe in hot water for a few days after childbirth.

A ceremonial bath is the major item of the menstrual rite of the Muthuvan girls. When a girl starts menstruation, her friends will take her to the nearby river in the morning of the coming day, and they spend hours there for taking a detailed bath. There is also a special bath in hot water after confinement. Some medicinal herbs are used while preparing hot water for the bath. The women may take bath in hot water for one or two weeks after confinement.

CLOTHING

The tribals predominantly wear cotton clothes. As there is no severe winter in this tract of the country, there is no need for woollen clothes. But as the nights are very cold in the higher elevations they sometimes use old sweaters or overcoats obtained from the planters or forest officials.

The men usually wear a loincloth and shirt. During summer they will not wear a shirt when engaged in work in the field. So the upper part of the body will be bare and receive sunrays and air abundantly. The Mannan women wear a 'Lungi' (a type of coloured loincloth) and blouse when they stay at home. They wear a saree when going out of the hamlet. The Muthuvan women always wear saree and blouse in their traditional style.

Often, the children upto two or three years go naked. They always play in the ground and move around with soiled body. The grown up male children wear either a loincloth or shorts. The school-going male children wear either shorts or loincloth and a shirt. The female children wear frock and blouse or shirt. They wear loincloth and long blouses while staying in the hamlet.

Some of the young Mannans have terrycotton pants and polyester shirts. They wear it while going to the town or during the festival season in the hamlet. A small percentage of the Mannan women have special night dress like gown.

The people use the same dress for three or four days and wash them afterwards using soap. One person may not have more than two pairs of dress. Many people wear the same dress in the night, which they have worn while working in the field during the day time. The old folk above 70 years of age, largely use their traditional dress.

HABITS OF EATING

There is some difference between the Muthuvans and Mannans with regard to the time of eating. The Muthuvans have only two important meals a day. They take it around 8 a.m. in the morning and by seven p.m. in the evening. So they have no lunch. They drink black tea during the interval. There is no special time for the intake of tea and they drink it whenever they want. Tea will be always ready in an aluminium pot, in a Muthuvan household.

The diet of the Muthuvans includes ragi, rice, pulses, tapioca, millets, vegetables, mushrooms, wild tubers, fruits etc. They cultivate ragi in the forest land and it forms their staple food. They dry the grains and take its flour by grinding it using a millstone. Then a thick, brownish paste is made by putting the flour in boiling water and kneading it thoroughly using a wooden spoon. This is known as 'katty' and is taken with some side dishes made of meat, fish or vegetables. They consume it immediately after cooking. When 'katty' is not available, they take rice. Rice is more costly as they have to purchase it from the market.

The Mannans take their chief meals two times a day. They take their meals at noon and around seven p.m. in the night. In the morning and in the afternoon they take either black coffee or black tea. The diet of the Mannans includes rice, ragi, millets, pulses, tapioca, wild tubers, vegetables green leaves, meat, fish, crabs, mushrooms etc. Their staple food is rice and is taken with a side dish prepared with some vegetables or flesh. Besides paddy they used to cultivate ragi and millets. But it will not be sufficient for them, for a whole year.

Due to deforestation and monoculture afforestation, the quality and variety of their diet has changed a lot. Now, most of the items of their traditional diet are not available in the forest. The ruthless destruction of natural forests and the afforestation programme consisting of foreign trees like Eucalyptus and Accacia adversely affect the availability of games, tubers, fruits, vegetables and mushrooms. So their present diet consists of rice, vegetables, pulses, wheat, meat and packed food like bread, biscuits, etc. This qualitative change of diet affects the intake of nutrients and is not adequate for their health.

The Muthuvans have some unhygienic eating habits. Very often two or more persons will eat from the same plate. Both elders and children follow this unhealthy practice. This unhygienic practice helps the spreading of contagious diseases. They eat from the same plate to show their friendship and group solidarity. But they are not aware of the ill effects of this practice.

LEAN PERIOD

The rainy season from June to August is a difficult period for the tribals. They cannot do any work in the field or go for any wage labour as there will be continuous rain during these months. Besides it is not the harvest period for crops like pepper, paddy, etc. So they suffer acute poverty during this period of time. Even hunger deaths are reported from the Mannans during this period in some years. As the tribals do not have the habit of saving for the future, they will be in real trouble when confronted with times of scarcity. Affliction of this acute poverty and starvation has its own adverse effect on the health of the tribals.

SPECIAL FOOD

Both the Muthuvans and Mannans provide some special food for women after confinement.

This food will generally continue for a few weeks after the birth of the child. The food includes medicinal herbs, vegetables, flesh of wild games like hog-deer, squirrel, porcupine etc., and a small quantity of liquor. The special food is provided to the women to regain the health and vitality, and also to produce more milk for the child. However they will not give any special food to the women when they are pregnant.

SOME ITEMS OF TRADITIONAL DIET

a. Tubers	b. Mushrooms	c. Honey	d. Liquor
Chon	Kumman		Aazha-
Thettom	Perumkoon		kallu.
Nuron	Pavakoon		
Kizhangu	Urumpukoon		

DRINKING HABITS

As mentioned earlier, coffee and tea are the common beverages used by the tribals. They do not mix milk in their beverages and in a way their intake of milk is very little. Either sugar or jaggery is used to sweeten the coffee or tea. But very often the poor folks may not be able to purchase sugar or jaggery and so they take the beverages without them.

The Muthuvans have an unhealthy practice while preparing tea. When the tea starts boiling, they will take a handful of cold water and sprinkle over the boiling tea. Then they dismount the tea-pot from the hearth. Often the water is taken without washing the hands and so this practice is very unhygienic. Secondly the tea will get cold and is not ideal for drinking. Thirdly if the water used for sprinkling is polluted, that will contaminate the tea. However, the Muthuvans sprinkle the cold water in order to send down the tea dust dancing in the boiling water. The sedimentation of the tea dust will be very quick after sprinkling the cold water.

SMOKING AND CHEWING

The Muthuvans are very fond of chewing *'pan'* and show only secondary interest in smoking *'beedi'* or cigarette. The *pan* includes a betel leaf, a piece of tobacco, a piece of arecanut and a little lime. Some people chew tobacco alone, without taking other ingredients of pan. Women also chew pan.

The Mannans have more affinity towards smoking and show only a secondary importance to chewing pan. They usually smoke *'beedi'* as it is more cheap. Whenever they have enough money, they will purchase cigarettes. Women never smoke, but a minority of them chew pan.

FOOD POLLUTION BY PETTY VENDORS

Even though the tribal hamlets are generally isolated in deep forests, the profit hungry petty vendors from small towns have no hesitation to overcome all these hurdles and reach the hamlets for selling their products. Most of their products are of cheap quality and they demand exorbitant prices for them. Food items are one of the important commodities usually brought by them. They sell a large variety of food substances like biscuits, lozenges, fried delicacies like banana chips and many other kinds of cheap sweetmeats.

They use materials of very low quality for the production of commodities to enhance their profit. For the tribals these spurious food items act as pollutants in their dietary habit.

SLEEPING HABITS

Both the Muthuvans and the Mannans sleep on the floor. Some wealthy Muthuvans use wooden cots while majority of them use a sack or a mat woven with the leaves of pandanus or grass. For the Mannans lying on a cot is a taboo.

Dormitory system is existing among the Muthuvans. The children and unmarried youth spend the night in separate male and female dormitories. In a dormitory children are sleeping very close to each other. Sick children are also sleeping in the dormitory which may pave the way for the spreading of diseases. People are not aware of this problem.

Usually the tribals go to sleep around 8 p.m. shortly after taking supper. The elders wake up by 5 a.m. while the children may sleep upto 6.30 a.m. As the hamlets are situated in high elevations, surrounded by the forest, the temperature is very low at night. So they put up a fire inside their house to quell the cold. As there are no windows for their houses the smoke will remain inside the room and slowly escape through the thatched roof. Breathing of this polluted air is not good for health. Some of the people have respiratory troubles and cough due to the continuous breathing of this smoke filled air. Many people have a burning sensation in the eyes. Now a days the Mannans generally discourage this habit and most of the younger people have stopped it. However, this is an effective mechanism to escape from the severe cold in the night.

DRINKS AND DRUGS

The tribals are very fond of drinking liquors like toddy, arrack, rum, brandy, etc. The Muthuvans know the technique to extract toddy known as *Aazhakallu* from a wild palm known as *Aazham.* It resembles the toddy obtained from the coconut tree in colour and taste. The toddy is extracted by making an incision in the spadix and a vessal will be tied under it, in such a position that the juice rinsing out of the spadix gets collected in it. The juice then gets fermented after a few hours and forms the toddy. Besides alcohol, the toddy contains a number of vitamins and is very nutritious.

The tribals drink both country-made arrack known as *Kottuvady* and also foreign liquors like brandy and rum. When they have money, a good part of it is wasted for drinking purposes. The tribals of some places know the technique to make arrack by the distillation process. They use articles like leech, old torch cells, ammonia, etc., to increase the quality of the *Kottuvady*. It will enhance the intoxication quality of the arrack, but is very harmful to health.

They drink large quantity of liquor during festivals or on other special occasions like marriage, puberty rites, etc. However, only few individuals are found as habitual drunkards. Most of them drink occasionally and it does not make any problem for their health.

Before they start drinking, a few drops of liquor will be offered to their gods. They will dip the forefinger in the liquor and offer three drops of liquor to gods. Otherwise the supernaturals may get angry with the people.

The tribals mainly smoke the inflorescence of the Indian hemp plant (Cannabis sativa) known as *Ganja* in their dialect. They cultivate the hemp plants around their houses which is also used as a medicine. They dry its inflorescence and insert this inside beedies or cigarettes and smoke. Sometimes tobacco will be mixed with this while smoking. A number of men in both communities are addicted to it. It is observed that it has adversely affected the health of people who use it daily. Some of the oldmen use opium also. Both tribes also smoke cigarettes ates his country-made cigarettes known as *beedi*.

The Table 5.1 shows the percentage of males in the Muthuvan and the Mannan community who have the vices of drinking and smoking ganja (hemp). As women rarely indulge in these unhealthy habits, they are not considered while taking these values.

Table 5.1 : Common Vices.

	Muthuvan	*Mannan*
Smoking Ganja (Hemp)	120 (24.43)	83 (15.09)
Drinking Liquor	143 (29.12)	196 (35.63)

DOMESTICATION OF ANIMALS

The Muthuvans and Mannans are not much interested in the domestication of animals. Only dogs are found in all their households. They are seen loitering even inside the houses and they sit close to their masters while they take food. Children consider them as their playmates. This over familiarity is not a healthy habit.

Cows and goats can be seen in a few houses as the people get loans from the Integrated Rural Development Programme (IRDP) for purchasing them. The Muthuvans usually keep the animals inside their houses at night. This is very unhygienic as the animals make the room filthy through defecation and the insects and ticks lodged in their hide can come to the people through close contact. They can disseminate various diseases to man.

The Mannans usually erect the cowshed close to their houses. This is to prevent the theft of animals and to protect them from the attack of wild animals. As the cowshed is so close to the house, the people always feel a stinking smell from there. A number of insects, flies, worms and mosquitoes breed in the open dung-pit. They can often function as carriers of different diseases.

A good percentage of tribals domesticate fowls. There may be a separate coop for them or they also may be kept inside the house in the night.

WATER SUPPLY AND SANITATION

The government has constructed water tanks in a limited number of hamlets and put up water taps for providing clean drinking water. In a few hamlets considerable reduction in the percentage of infant mortality was noticed after providing safe drinking water. So the people have a positive attitude towards the installation of water taps in their hamlets.

However, they do not know how to use the water economically and keep the surroundings of the water tap clean. In most of the places, there is no cemented base around the water tap. So the water from the tap always falls on the ground and a mire-pit is often developed around the tap. The problem is more serious if the tap is a leaking one. People use to waste a lot of water by not closing the taps after use, and the children play with it very often. "The provision of water supply and basic sanitation facilities would not automatically improve health. The availability of such facilities should be accompanied by intensive health education campaigns for the improvement of personal hygiene, the economic use of water and the sanitary disposal of waste in a manner that will improve individual and community health." (Statement on National Health Policy, 1982).

In some hamlets, the water taps are found dry during summer. Some of the water sources get dried up during this season. However, the need of tap water is more during summer as there are more chances of water pollution at that time.

CONCEPT OF HEALTH

The tribals have no clear concepts about health. A person is considered healthy when he is not afflicted by any disease, consumes food as usual and carries out his normal functions without any difficulty. When somebody is sick, they will employ all efforts to heal his illness and bring him back to normal condition. However, there is no effort to prevent the occurrence of diseases by keeping personal hygiene and preserving sanitary environment.

In the past they completely depended upon the forest for food and medicine. The forest produces like honey, tubers, fruits, etc., and the flesh of various games were very nutritious and ideal for good health. They have obtained a number of medicinal plants also from the forest which could heal their diseases. Since they subsisted on forest produces, there was no problem of adulteration or food pollution. The deforestation and monoculture afforestation with trees like Eucalyptus, Teak (Tectona grandis), etc. tilted the balance of their natural habitat. The foreign trees like Eucalyptus and Acacia suck all the underground water and the wells and other water sources get dried up. This new forest is not able to provide produces like honey, tubers, fruits, etc. Availability of games also has decreased. There is a dearth of medicinal plants also. The poor condition of the forests tends the tribals to look for marketed food articles and the modern medicinal system.

The change that occurred in the quality of diet has an adverse effect on the health of the tribals. For the first time they have experienced the evils like adulteration, pollution, etc., which have a telling effect on their health. This paves the way for the origin of new diseases among them. Their traditional medicineman is helpless to cure this new type of diseases. The forest environment today is no more a healthy retreat and the tribals are paying for it at the cost of their health.

PATIENT'S APPROACH TOWARDS DISEASE CONDITION

Generally the tribals do not give much attention to a disease situation. They consider it a shameful thing to lie on somewhere for a minor ailment. Their unfriendly habitat tends them to do hardwork for getting food. So, only when somebody is seriously ill, will he lie down and take rest. Then it is the responsibility of his family members to look after him and to provide necessary treatment.

COMMUNITY'S ATTITUDE TOWARDS A PATIENT

The Muthuvans are generally indifferent towards a patient. If the disease is a contagious one, they will isolate the person and abandon him in a separate house. Minimum attention will be given to him afterwards.

Sick children can be seen lying on a mat covered with a cloth in the corner of the house. Parents will give him food and medicine at intervals. When they go out, the child will be left alone in the house. In the past they used to abandon all the patients when any epidemic broke out, and leave that hamlet and go to a new dwelling place. In the present age they will try all their ethnomedicine for various ailments.

The Mannans show more attention to the patients. Children are never left alone in a house, but somebody will be always there to look after the sick children. They also do not go for medicine when affected by some minor ailments. They may either take some home remedies or simply take rest. Still they depend upon their ethnomedicine for the treatment of a number of diseases. If it can not bring cure, then the patient may be taken to a hospital.

RELIGIOUS BELIEFS AND HEALTH

For the tribals religion plays an important role in all spheres of their life. Even in health care religious beliefs and practices have their own specific influence. Because of the lack of proper health education they derive the cause of many of the diseases from religious teachings. Thus the supernatural forces play a direct role in the causation and cure of many of the diseases. The medicinemen of the community act as mediators between the people and the supernatural powers. They make offerings to the deities and ancestral spirits on behalf of the patients.

The tribals believe that a cordial relationship with the deities and ancestral spirits will ensure good health for the members of the community. So, they perform various ceremonies every year during the annual festivals, to renovate their relationship with the supernaturals, and thus ensure the protection of the hamlet. Viswanathan Nair has observed: "most of the annual ancestral propitiation ceremonies can be considered as ventures to ensure proper health of the society" (1985:341). They also believe that if proper propitiation is not offered to the deities and to ancestral spirits, then they will get angry and send diseases and other calamities to the members of the community.

MEDICAL PLURALISM

In the past there was only ethnomedicine to deal with all kinds of illness situations in the tribal communities. Health has been regulated in such traditional communities by the medicineman or shaman, on the basis of sound ecological factors, although neither the healer nor the patient may have been consciously aware of the underlying basis of treatment. The medicineman derives all his medicines from the nature, which includes both plant parts, animal matter and minerals. As medicines are the products from the forest, there is no degenerating effect. All the medicines come from the environment to which the tribal community has adapted themselves.

With the passing of time major changes have occurred in their habitat. Large portions of natural forest were destroyed and were replaced by monoculture plantations of Eucalyptus, Teak, Acacia, etc. The influx of non-tribals from the plains resulted in more contact with modern culture. The scarcity of food inside the forest tended the tribals to seek food from outside world.

By the middle of this century, the government has started a number of hospitals, health centres and dispensaries in the tribal areas to improve the health of the tribal people. The change of diet and living conditions gradually led to the origin of a number of new diseases among them, for which the ethnomedicine has no answer. After getting some education and experiencing the advantages of modern medicine, the tribals have started using modern medicine for the treatment of new diseases.

Thus more than one type of medical system came into practice in the tribal universe. This new innovation created numerous problems in the tribal communities. The philosophy and practice of modern medicine was alien to them.

The policy of government to uplift the health condition of tribals through the introduction of modern medicine has a number of good as well as bad impacts on the tribals. Many of them first rejected this new system of medicine. But with the passage of time, they have slowly started accepting it for the treatment of certain diseases. Age, economic status, isolation from nontribals, spatial mobility, sex, education, etc., are some of the factors influencing the selection of medicine. But the modern medicine often could not satisfy all their needs. So, most of the people are now using the more efficacious elements of both systems of medicine. They select a particular kind of medicine according to the nature and seriousness of their illness.

CHOICE OF MEDICINE

In the selection of medicine no clear preference towards any system could not be noticed. They avail the facilities of both types of medicine according to the nature of illness. The diseases originating from supernatural causes are always treated by the traditional medicineman. Economic constraints and the sylvan isolation very often deter the people from using modern medicine. The results obtained from the household health survey show that ethnomedicine has a definite edge on modern medicine. Among the Muthuvans who are more tradition-oriented this difference is more clear. While a good percentage of people show no preference for any system of medicine.

Table 5.2 : Preference for Medicine

	Muthuvan	*Mannan*	*Total*
Ethnomedicine	116 (58.0)	78 (39.0)	194 (48.50)
Modern medicine	43 (21.50)	70 (35.0)	113 (28.25)
No preference	41 (20.50)	52 (26.0)	93 (23.25)
Total	200	200	400

Figures In the parentheses denote percentage.

ECONOMIC CONSTRAINTS AND MODERN MEDICINE

Economic constraints form a major hurdle in availing the benefits of modern medicine. People are found struggling to purchase even rice, teapowder and other essential commodities during the lean period. When somebody gets sick in this period, they depend upon ethnomedicine for cure. The patient may survive if the treatment is successful, otherwise he may die. The summer season is a vulnerable period and several epidemics break out during this time. Without getting proper care and effective medicine many people die. Scarcity of drinking water, unhygienic surroundings, hostile climate and inability to go for modern medicine increase the death rate.

CULTURAL BARRIERS AND MODERN MEDICINE

As the tribals belong to a special culture, they have some difficulty to mingle with the people of other cultures. All the medical personnel are members of the non-tribal culture. While undergoing treatment a close interaction is necessary between the members of both cultures. The cultural barrier was a major hurdle in the successful implementation of medical programmes. But now, the seriousness of this problem has been considerably decreased due to greater interaction between the tribals and the nontribals.

However, this problem is still existing among the Muthuvan women. They enjoy less freedom and always the menfolk have an eye on their movements. So, the Muthuvan women rarely visit hospitals for treatment. They may be either treated by the medicineman of the community or their husbands or parents get medicine for them from hospitals. Confinement takes place in the hamlet always under the supervision of a few old ladies.

Table 5.3 : Attendance at the time of confinement

	Muthuvan	*Mannan*	*Total*
Traditional midwife/old women in the neighbourhood	34	22	56
Hospital	1	4	5
Total	35	26	61

The Mannan women enjoy more freedom than their Muthuvan counterparts. However, most of them are availing the services of traditional midwives and other old women during the time of their delivery. Their reluctance to mingle with the non-tribal medical personnel, taboos against the presence of a male at the time of confinement and the economic constraints are the major reasons which motivate the women to give birth to their children at home.

NON-AVAILABILITY OF MODERN MEDICINE

The non-availability of modern medicine is one of the major reasons for the continuous use of ethnomedicine. The Muthuvans living in remote areas like *Edamalakudy* and the Mannans living in the interior places like *Variyam* have to walk 20 to 30 kilometres to reach a hospital. There is no road and the jungle path passing through steep hills and rocky cliffs is not good enough for a sickman to go to a hospital. Therefore, when somebody is sick in such interior areas, he will approach the shaman or medicineman of the hamlet and follow his treatment.

In some cases there is combined use of both modern and ethnomedicine. When a patient is very weak and cannot go to hospital by foot, he will take ethnomedicine from the healer of the hamlet. After a few days' treatment there may be some relief in his condition and he may be able to move around without difficulty. Then he will go to a hospital in the nearby town and undergo treatment there, for getting a complete and speedy cure. Thus people select the type of medicine according to their need and pressure of circumstances.

CHOICE OF HOSPITALS

The tribals show a marked preference for private hospitals over government ones. According to some Muthuvans, the government hospitals are places to kill the patients. One who wants to die can go there and undergo the free treatment available there. The Mannans also hold similar views.

The major reasons put forward by the tribals in the selection of hospitals are:-

1. In government hospitals nobody will show any interest towards the patients, and they have to wait for a long time for getting service and medicine. The attitude of doctors, nurses and other officials is very indifferent. According to some Mannans, the government want more people to die daily because when one man dies, the government can save the rice and other food stuffs needed for that person.

2. The medicines available from the government hospitals are very poor in quality. In many cases, medicines are not available and the tribals have to buy them from outside.

3. For getting good medicine and care the patients have to bribe the doctors and other officials.

4. In the private hospital doctors and the nurses show interest towards the patients and listen to their complaints patiently. This cordial approach gives much relief to them.

5. Even though they have to pay money for the medicine and stay, the patients can get good, efficacious medicine from private hospitals. So they do not bother about spending money in a private hospital rather than go to a

government hospital where they will not get any care or good medicine.

The premises of government hospitals are very unhygienic. The private hospitals and their premises are better than the government hospitals. But they are also far below satisfactory level. The rooms are often crowded and in some seasons the patients will not get even a bed and will have to lie down on the floor.

Purchasing medicines directly from the chemist of the medical shop and their self-administration is another practice prevailing among the tribals. People are not aware of the dangers embedded in this habit.

MEDICAL TEAMS AND THEIR EFFECTIVENESS

Epidemics used to break out every year in the tribal hamlets during the summer and rainy seasons. Chickenpox, measles, cholera, diarrhoea, whooping cough, etc., are the common maladies affecting them. Usually the outside world will come to know of the onset of epidemics only very slowly as most of the tribal hamlets are situated inside dense forests in remote places. Very often news about the outbreak of epidemics reaches the outer world late and through merchants and newspaper reporters visiting the tribal area. When news come in the dailies, the concerned government departments will suddenly become active and medical teams consisting of doctors, nurses and pharmacists will be sent to the tribal hamlets for distributing medicine to the needy patients. But, by the time the medical teams reach the hamlets, a number of patients would have passed away.

The response of the Mannans is very positive towards medical teams. They accept medicines from the doctors and consume them for the cure of diseases.

However, the response of the Muthuvans towards medical teams is often negative. They believe that epidemics like measles and cholera originate by some supernatural causes. So no medicine is effective in checking them. If they take any medicine that will aggravate the anger of god and consequently the disease also will get serious. To avoid this unpleasant development, they will tell the medical personnel that nobody is sick in their house and they do not need any medicine. The Muthuvan women and children are very shy to face the outsiders and often they will run away when the medical team approaches a hamlet.

So, only through much persuasion and threat, will the Muthuvans come forward to get themselves examined by the doctor and to receive the medicine. But, the treatment of disease using force is often ineffective because there is no way to know whether they will consume the medicine provided to them. With a short visit the medical personnel cannot enlighten them about the efficacy of modern medicine. So the effort to thrust upon modern medicine within a short time span will make them suspicious and they may react towards it in a negative manner.

As the Muthuvans firmly believe that the cause of the epidemic is the anger of god, in their view it is illogical and harmful for the patient to take any kind of medicine. Only after removing this hurdle through imparting proper health education, can the medical team expect a positive response from them. Very often it is found that the Muthuvans simply waste the medicines supplied to them by keeping them somewhere in the house.

DRAWBACKS OF MEDICAL TEAM

The visit of medical teams during the outbreak of epidemics has a number of handicaps. The absence of rapport between the doctors and the tribals is a hindrance in giving modern medicine to them. The doctor is a strange person for them, and the tribals by their very nature will not trust strangers. The medical personnel are also discouraged by the non-cooperative attitude of the tribals.

The most important drawback Is that there will be no follow-up visits or treatment after the visit. So the patients will not get medicine and care till their illness is completely cured. If a person who takes medicine from the medical team cannot get any relief because of the lack of availability of a full course of medicine, he will be discouraged to take it again in future.

AYURVEDIC DISPENSARY AND THE TRIBALS

To improve the standard of health of the tribals, government agencies like, Integrated Tribal Development Project (ITDP) have started a few ayurvedic dispensaries in some tribal settlements. In the tribal hamlet of 'Korangatty colony' at Adimaly an ayurvedic dispensary is functioning with a doctor and a pharmacist. The tribal communities found in the *'Korangatty colony'* are

'Mala Arayans', 'Ulladans', 'Mannans' and *'Muthuvans'*. All of them are not found exploiting the facilities available in the dispensary in the same manner.

The duty doctor revealed that the percentage of 'Ulladans' and 'Mala Arayans' is very high among the patients. Mannans are also taking ayurvedic medicines to a limited extent, even though they have their own ethnomedicine. However, the Muthuvans are most reluctant in visiting the dispensary for treatment. After receiving medicine free of cost they may sometimes keep it in their homes without giving it to the patients.

The doctor has also noticed that the Muthuvans are showing particular interest towards certain types of medicines when they visit the dispensary. They evaluate the efficacy of medicines by noting its colour and taste. They like certain reddish *'Arishtam'* and *'Lehyam'* while they show much hesitation in consuming the *'Kashayam'* (a medicinal decoction) which is actually very effective in checking diseases. But the interesting thing is that, the same persons who refused to take *'Kashayam'* for fever, will demand it when they have some skin diseases like scabies or itches.

Thus the Muthuvans like to take their own decisions in the selection of medicines according to the nature of various diseases. They are not blind followers of the advice given by the doctor, but consider their own previous experiences with each kind of medicine. So, the doctor is compelled to play a passive role while treating the Muthuvan patients.

DOCTOR-PATIENT RELATIONSHIP

The communication between the doctor and the patient is not often satisfactory. The patient sometimes fails to convey the details of the symptoms properly or gives overemphasis to any one of them. Some of the patients may not be able to understand the method of medication ordered by the doctor.

Often the doctors consider the tribals as ignorant people having a number of superstitions and do not give any seriousness to their disease causation beliefs. It is found that the patients always like the doctors who have some knowledge in their concepts of etiology and treatment. They claim that some of the doctors have told them that for the cure of certain diseases the help of god is necessary and making offerings to god is an appropriate act.

But some of the doctors are very busy and they will not ask any personal questions to their patients. His inquiry will be limited to the disease only. People do not have much enthusiasm to follow the directions of such doctors. Often the doctors in the government hospitals belong to this category. The doctors of private hospitals spend more time with each patient and try to become friendly to him by asking many personal questions, which may not be often relevant for the treatment of illness. The tribals have much appreciation about this type of doctors and they contact them again when affected by a disease. Some of the doctors in the private hospitals may even give some concessions in the cost of treatment, or allow the tribals to pay the money in convenient instalments.

CO-OPERATION OF PATIENTS IN THE TREATMENT

After contacting a doctor and receiving medicines from him, there are many other factors in the successful completion of the treatment. Because of the lack of education and limited experience with modern medicine the tribal patients often make mistakes in the treatment procedure. Before taking a patient to the hospital, most of the tribals will try their ethnomedicine. In some cases they may bring the patient to the hospital in a critical stage. So it is, more difficult for the doctor to treat such cases.

Most of the allopathic medicines have to be taken at specific intervals for checking the disease successfully. The tribals often make mistakes in taking the medicines on time and in the right quantity. Sometimes when they go out for work, they may skip their doses. All these make the use of modern medicine ineffective.

Usually the tribals are satisfied with a symptomatic relief and show much reluctance to come back to the hospital for continuing the treatment. This hesitation to visit the doctor for the follow-up treatment may prevent complete cure and lead to the return of the disease. An illness prolonging for a long time will be then considered as having originated due to the wrath of god.

The tribals are least bothered about following the advice of the doctor like diet control, taking rest and avoiding hardwork, smoking and drinking. They will not take rest unless they are so weak to do any work. Actually they do not know the relevance of these restrictions and their interrelationship with the treatment. The treatment will not be effective when the patient violates the advice of the doctor. Then the doctor and his medicines may be considered as incapable of healing the illness.

DOUBLE-DEALING OF SHAMANS

The shamans belonging to the Mannan community adopt a double standard in evaluating the efficacy of modern medicine in the treatment of diseases. Publicly they will criticize modern medicine and opine that after curing one illness, it may cause another one. They seem to have some crude idea about the side effects of modern medicine. They will also praise the efficacy of ethnomedicine and explain to their clients how it is suitable for the human body. They may sometimes ridicule the folly of people who seek modern medicine for the cure of illness.

But the strange fact is that when these shamans are affected by some disease very often they will go to a hospital or purchase medicine directly from the medical shop. Often they try to hide from others that they are getting treatment from the hospitals. So they may contact the doctors in the far away hospitals. This shows the double dealing of the Mannan shamans while evaluating the efficacy of modern medicine.

FAMILY WELFARE

Only a small percentage of men and women in the reproductive age have taken permanent method of sterilization. People have many prejudices and misconceptions about this method of family planning. They consider that vasectomy and tubectomy are detrimental to health and would cause backache and fatigue. This will affect their ability to engage in hardwork.

Some of their complaints may be psychological, arising out of a fear towards surgery. However, many of the complaints may have a genuine physiological cause behind them. Most of the people are undergoing vasectomy during the camps organized by the Family Welfare Department. The acceptors do not get proper care or attention during such busy programmes. As the doctors have to carry out so many operations a day, they cannot be much careful with each person. Due to the hurry in the work they may commit some mistakes.

Besides, the poor tribals are not in a position to take enough rest after the operation. Their poor living conditions compel them to engage in hardwork from the next day onwards. This lack of aftercare also may be a reason for the origin of complaints among those who have undergone the contraceptive surgery.

Table 5.4 : Acceptance of Family Welfare Measures

	Muthuvan	Mannan	Total
Vasectomy	12	52	64
Tubectomy	17	74	91
Total	29	126	155

The monetary incentive is the main reason for undergoing the surgical operation. Five cases are noticed among the Mannans where both husband and wife are found to be subjected to the contraceptive surgery because of the offer of incentives.

PROPHYLACTIC MEASURES

The tribals are not aware of the relevance of preventive measures in the modern medicine for escaping from the diseases. They do not voluntarily take preventive injections for any disease. Some of the tribals got preventive injections as a part of the immunisation programme of the government. But the people living in the remote areas are not often covered by these programmes.

In their day-to-day life the tribals do not take any special care for the prevention of diseases. They have some supernatural measures like wearing of amulet, offering of sacrifices to god, etc., which are believed to be capable of preventing illnesses. "Undoubtedly in many situations magical resources may also be prophylactically effective. In a society where belief in magical attacks may induce severe stress that can lead to illness and death, reliance on the protection of an amulet may be psychically hygienic" (Lieban, 1973:1046).

The tribals are not much aware of the relevance of personal hygiene and environmental sanitation in the prevention of diseases. Actually they are not in a position to improve their living conditions due to socio-economic backwardness. According to Matthews, "when people do not have even the minimum necessities, it is hard for them to appreciate the value of preventive measures which will bring only probable benefits in the future" (1978:261).

Table 5.5 : Acceptance of Prophylactic measures

	Muthuvan	*Mannan*
Vaccination	123 (12.36)	309 (27.91)
DTP	23 (2.31)	61 (5.51)
BCG	Nil	14 (1.26.)

Figures in the parentheses denote percentage.

REASONS FOR THE SURVIVAL OF ETHNOMEDICINE

Ethnomedicine is still persisting in the tribal communities even after the introduction of modern medicine since a number of decades. Of course, its former popularity and reliability has considerably eroded and a number of tribals are now exploiting the facilities of modern medicine in addition to ethnomedicine. However, through a close observation one can find out that traditional ethnomedicine is still viable and it plays a commendable role in the treatment of ailments among the tribals. A detailed analysis in the following pages will explain the favourable factors for the survival of this system of medicine.

1. Easy Availability

At present the majority of curative centres like hospitals, dispensaries, etc., are located in urban areas. So the people seeking medical assistance have to travel long distances to reach the nearest hospital. The tribals often do not have either the resources or the ability to go to the hospitals in the urban areas. So they look forward to ethnomedicine which is easily available in their own locality for protecting them from the ailments.

2. Economy

The tribals have to spend a lot of money for getting efficient treatment from the private hospitals. Only cheap medicines are available from the government hospitals. For most of the costly medicines the doctors will give prescription notes and the patients have to buy them from the medical stores outside the hospital. Most of the tribals cannot afford this treatment. So they depend upon ethnomedicine which is available free of cost. The medicineman do not demand any money and all the medicines are available from nature.

3. Efficacy

Ethnomedicine is very efficacious in checking a number of diseases. The magico-religious therapy of shaman is aided by the powerful tool of suggestion, which is very helpful in bringing about cure. The rituals of shamans have much psychological impact upon the patient and he believes that the efficient techniques of shaman can remove his illness.

The plant, animal and mineral matters used in the drug therapy of ethnomedicine have real physicotherapeutic effect upon the patients. The tribals have a rich knowledge about the medicinal properties of various plants and they use them effectively in the treatment of diseases. In addition to this, they have other techniques like diet control, fasting, massage, bone-setting, etc., to face various types of ailments.

4. Purity

Most of the tribals opine that ethnomedicine is harmless and more suitable for the body. As plant, mineral and animal materials obtained from nature are used for the preparation of medicine, its function inside the body will be quite natural and rejuvenating. They hold the belief that even though modern medicine gives quick relief, it is harmful to the body. After healing one illness, the harmful principles of the medicine can cause another disease in the same person sometime later.

5. Screening

It is found that when both ethno and modern medicines are available the patients or their relatives take some arbitrary decisions about what kind of medicine is suitable for the treatment of a particular disease. Often they approach the medicineman for minor ailments and go to a hospital for serious diseases. In some cases the medicineman will carry out a second screening. After examining the patient, he will send the more complicated cases to a hospital. It is known as the "remittance function" of the indigenous practitioner (Djurfeldt and Lindberg, 1976:178).

As a result of screening, modern medicine will get the more complicated and serious cases while ethnomedicine will get only cases of minor illnesses. So, the percentage of success will be higher in the case of ethnomedicine than in the case of modern medicine. Thus the screening is favourable to the ethnomedicine and contributes to its apparent efficiency.

6. Healer-Patient Relationship

The practitioner of ethnomedicine is an insider to the community and the patients have personal relationships with him. The healer is related to the patient as a friend, kinsman, etc. So their relationship is very cordial and informal. After diagnosis, the medicinemen will explain to the patient the causes and remedies of the illness. Thus, along with the healer, the patient also has an active role in the treatment procedure. This will ensure full co-operation of the patient with the healer and their joint effort will bring success easily.

The relationship between a patient and a doctor is formal and they are representatives of two different cultures. The doctor will ask a number of questions to the patient about the disease and seldom explain the cause and remedy of the illness. The interest of the doctor in the patient is limited to the disease, its diagnosis and treatment.

THE WEAKNESSES OF MODERN MEDICINE IN THE TRIBAL UNIVERSE

Even though modern medicine was introduced in the tribal communities a number of decades ago, it can not still attain the monopoly of health care among them. It plays only a complementary role along with ethnomedicine. Even today, for the treatment of certain diseases the tribals prefer their own ethnomedicine to the modern one. The inherent weaknesses of the modern medical system and the resistance of ethnomedicine to it are the two most important reasons for the partial success of modern medicine.

U.N. Dhebar (1961) has pointed out four reasons for the shortfall in implementing the programmes for tribal medical services.

1. The need for correct approach.
2. Problem of personnel.
3. Inadequacy of communications.
4. Rules about supply of medicine.

Shortage of sufficient number of doctors and qualified nurses is the greatest handicap of allopathic hospitals. The doctors and nurses are much reluctant, to work in the tribal areas. After being posted in such places they will try to get a transfer from there as early as possible. Often they may not come to the hospital regularly. The living conditions are very poor in the tribal areas and no facilities of urban life are available there. Problems of housing, recreation, education of children, contact with the outside world, etc., are the common difficulties in such places.

Lack of an adequate infrastructure is another hurdle facing modern medicine. Often there may not be good buildings, beds, vehicles, laboratories, X-ray units and other essential hospital equipment for the hospitals and Primary Health Centres functioning in the tribal areas. The doctors are much dissatisfied due to this adverse circumstances and sometimes they may fail to diagnose the diseases correctly. These disadvantages adversely affect the quality of medical treatment available in these curative centres. Inadequate supply of medicines is another serious handicap. The patients will be discouraged to go to the hospital when medicine is not available there.

The prejudice of tribal patients to accept wholly the modern medicine is also a hurdle, hindering its widespread recognition. The medicinemen and shamans often resent modern medical programmes because they fear that the competition will be injurious to their status in the community.

6

Conclusion: Change and Adaptation of Ethnomedicine

In the present study an attempt has been made to describe the ethnomedical system of the Muthuvans and the Mannans not as a set of abstract beliefs and exotic practices, or in isolation, but as an essential part of the tribal social structure. As the various ethnomedical beliefs and practices are closely interrelated with the social organization, religious beliefs and life crises, due attention has been given to each one of them. Since the different components of social structure are closely connected with each other, an analysis of one aspect needs an understanding of the remaining aspects also.

The Muthuvans and the Mannans possess some similarities as both of them live in similar habitats and on identical tracts of the forest. The dietary habits of both communities bear a number of similar features. Barring these few similarities, both communities show differences in culture, tradition, religious beliefs, social structure, dialect and level of acculturation.

Ethnomedicine, being an important social system, also follows these similarities and dissimilarities. Both tribal communities have a rich knowledge of ethnomedicine and depend upon it for their health care. Magic and herbal therapy are the two basic components of ethnomedicine of both groups. As the 'materia medica' are collected from the same habitat there are a number of common remedies present in both communities. However, their magical rituals are entirely different and in this field no transfer of knowledge has taken place. Each group preserved its own divination techniques, spells, curing rituals and prophylactic measures as the sole property of the community. As knowledge in the magical practices is accessible to only a few selected persons in both groups, they could keep them as top secrets and treat them as the most valuable treasure of the community.

The Muthuvans and the Mannans have been exposed to modern medicine in the same period. As the Muthuvans are living in more remote places than the Mannans, the influence of modern medicine was less among them. Some variations also can be seen in the ways the two communities reacted towards this external influence. Both communities did not accept modern medicine in the early stages of its implementation. But their negative attitude was changed with the passage of time. However, it can be noticed that the Mannans are more enthusiastic in exploiting the facilities of modern medicine, while the Muthuvans are accepting it reluctantly and also due to the pressure of circumstances.

With the large-scale immigration of non-tribals from the plains, a lot of changes have occurred in the High Ranges which is the abode of these tribals. The land-hungry and hard working non-tribals have converted large areas of forests into agricultural fields and plantations. They have introduced the cultivation of various cash crops like rubber, pepper, tea, cardamom, lemongrass, ginger, etc. Often they have grabbed the land of the tribals and driven them to the interior areas of forests.

Various government agencies also have played an important role in the alteration of the habitat of this region. The Kerala State Electricity Board constructed a few dams in this area for generating hydroelectric power. The Idukki dam constructed across the river 'Periyar' is the biggest one, which is also the highest archdam in Asia. Construction of these dams caused the displacement of a large number of tribals from their catchment areas. Besides, these hydroelectric projects paved the way for the destruction of large areas of the natural forest. The Kerala State Forest Department also gave large areas of forest land to the private contractors for clearfelling. This was to increase the revenue of the state. After clearfelling, the Government has replaced the forest by monoculture plantations of Teak, Eucalyptus, Acacia, Pine, etc. These plantations have no resemblance to the natural forest, it had displaced.

This change of habitat adversely affected the life of the tribals. After large-scale deforestation they could not get the traditional items of food from the forest. They are confronted with the scarcity of medicinal plants and animal matter also. For the first time in their history they have been exposed to the vices of adulteration and pollution. After the contact with non-tribals and also due to the change in consumption pattern, new diseases came into existence among them. Most of these diseases were unknown to them in the past. So the tribal medicinemen find it difficult to treat these new diseases. At this juncture, modern medicine has played a crucial role. When the tribals found that their ethnomedicine is ineffective in curing the new diseases, some of them sought the assistance of modern medicine. From their experience, they have realized that modern medicine is very efficient in healing the new ailments. However, even after they have started using modern medicine, ethnomedicine has continued to play a significant role in the health care of the tribals. They have used both systems of medicine according to the nature of disease etiology and mode of treatment.

SOME DRAWBACKS OF ETHNOMEDICINE

The knowledge about ethnomedicine is a part of the traditional lore of the community. This secret knowledge about medicinal plants and magical rituals are always transferred orally through generations and there are no written documents to store this knowledge.

The ethnomedical system of the present age is in a more or less static condition. Research and development are concepts which are unknown to the tribal medicinemen. They follow the age-old medicinal combinations and healing techniques which they have inherited from their forefathers.

This medical system is a closed one and it is neither experimental nor does it imbibe any knowledge from other cultures in any systematic way.

Ethnomedicine often cannot cope with the fast changes occurring in the community. Changes occurred in the habitat, subsistence pattern and dietary habits of the tribals and the close association with non-tribals tilted the balance of their traditional life. Along with these changes acculturation brought forth many new diseases to them. Most of these diseases were not present among them in the past and hence the tribal medicinemen are helpless to tackle them. It is quite natural that there is no medicine for maladies like pollution and adulteration in nature. The medicinemen are not able to diagnose these causes which are not familiar to them.

The medicinemen of present age are not as competent as their predecessors. As the tribals in the past solely depended upon the forest for their food and medicine, the medicinemen of those ages had a vast knowledge of the medicinal properties of flora and fauna. Especially the Mannans gradually lost their close familiarity with the forest, when they changed their subsistence pattern from shifting cultivation to settled agriculture. With the death of the old medicinemen, considerable amount of knowledge was lost to the community. There are also some professional hindrances which retarded the passing of medical knowledge from a medicineman to his disciples. It is a commonly accepted notion that no teacher must teach all his techniques to his disciples. So the teachers used to hold back some of the important techniques from the disciples in order to keep up his supremacy. Some of the teachers want to reveal this knowledge in their last days. But very often they will not get any opportunity to do so and the precious medical knowledge will be lost for ever.

Deforestation plays a role disadvantageous to the ethnomedical system. The large-scale destruction of natural forest adversely affected both flora and fauna of this part of the country. A number of medicinal plants have been destroyed by the ruthless denudation of forest and today the medicinemen suffer from the scarcity of these plants. As the tribals do not have the habit of growing medicinal plants for their needs, they have always depended upon natural sources. When these natural sources are destroyed they find it difficult to collect the various essential ingredients of medicinal preparations. This is equally applicable in the case of animals also. They used to mix a number of animal matter as ingredients of medicines. But deforestation affected their availability also.

The expertise of tribal medicinemen in the art of surgery is very crude and not sufficient for the successful treatment of complicated cases. Even though they have a good knowledge in the bone-setting technique, they may commit mistakes when fractures are involved. Due to the mistakes in the treatment some of the patients are found handicapped.

The sceptical attitude of the patients is a new problem confronting the practitioners of ethnomedicine. After getting little education and experiencing the capacity of modern medicine to impart speedy relief, the tribals, especially the youngsters, are more sceptical towards the capability of ethnomedical practices. This disbelief often retard the pace of the healing process. When the cure come very slowly the patients may go to a hospital for availing the facilities of modern medicine for a speedy relief. This problem is more serious among the Mannan patients who have close association with the nontribals.

Now a days some of the Mannans are using ethnomedicine as a stopgap arrangement. When they cannot easily get modern medicine they depend upon ethnomedicine as the only medical facility available on the spot. But, afterwards, they will go to the modern curative centres for further treatment. To cite an example, when somebody gets sick in the night or when he is inside the dense forest, there is no question of getting modern medicine immediately. So he will quickly resort to ethnomedicine which is available easily. If the illness persists, he will go to a hospital on the next day or when he could come out of the forest. So, such people have more belief in the quick relief brought by modern medicine and use ethnomedicine only as a stopgap arrangement.

After the advent of modern medicine, the Mannans and also the Muthuvans living in the border areas of forests, used to take arbitrary decisions, based on their previous experiences, about what kind of disease is to be taken to which type of practitioners for treatment. Generally they show preference for the modern curative centres when afflicted by serious ailments and are satisfied with ethnomedicine for the treatment of minor illnesses and also maladies originating due to assumed supernatural causes. After reducing the use of ethnomedicine for treatment of minor illnesses, it lost its prestige value and popular appeal as an efficient medical system. However, the Muthuvans living in dense forests do not take such arbitrary decisions and are availing the facilities of ethnomedicine for all their ailments.

INTRODUCTION OF MODERN MEDICINE: ITS IMPACT ON THE COMMUNITY

The introduction of modern medicine has multiple impact on the community in general and ethnomedical system in particular. This is a new system of medicine and all its methods and concepts of etiology are alien to them. In the initial stage (Phase-1) of its introduction, nobody bothered to avail its facilities, as people thought that it was not ideal for their culture and was not able to treat their illness. So, this phase was a period of non contact between the community and modern medicine. In this phase they continued the use of ethnomedicine for the treatment of illnesses afflicting them. Because of the withdrawal of the tribals, modern medicine could not do anything worthwhile for the health care of the tribals in its initial period of existence in the tribal areas.

However, with the passage of time the tribals started availing the facilities of modern medicine (Phase-II). The efforts of the medical personnel, spread of education, increased mobility, close association with nontribal immigrants, etc., influenced the way of thinking of the tribals and helped them to use modern medicine. Initially, the use of modern medicine by a small percentage of the people evoked a rebellious attitude among the rest of the community. Often the elders and medicinemen ridiculed the people who used modern medicine which, in their opinion, was useless.

But the people who used modern medicine found it efficacious and capable of bringing speedy relief. Their favourable experience attracted others also who were sceptical to it earlier. So, in the course of time, more people started using this new system of therapy. Actually these people were ignorant of the underlying principles of modern medicine and of the ideas behind its mode of treatment. They were simply attracted by the curative ability of modern medicine.

Even in this phase of transition people believe in supernatural causes for certain diseases. They believe that some diseases originated from the supernatural reasons like evil eye, sorcery, breach of taboo, anger of ancestral spirits and wrath of god. For the treatment of such diseases they are still depending upon ethnomedicine. While, for certain other illnesses like chickenpox, measles and cholera they do not take any medicine at all because of the reasons stated earlier in chapter six. Even if some modern medical help is resorted to, they are not of much help in curing diseases like chickenpox and measles. So, the modern medical practitioner cannot eradicate the superstition that smallpox and chickenpox are due to the wrath of '*Mariyamma*'. Gould made it clear that, "modern medicines have very little effect as a matter of fact once a person contracts smallpox. Consequently the modern medical practitioner is not able to counter the powerful religious aversions to treatment with a powerful cure of his own" (1965:205).

After prolonged experience with modern medicine the tribals have realized (Phase-III) that, there is no miracle attached to its treatment and that it is not capable of healing every illness with equal effectiveness. They have also found that for the cure of certain illnesses their own ethnomedicine is more efficient than the modern one. So, gradually they have started selecting the type of medicine according to the nature of the illness. Without blindly following a certain mode of treatment, they have utilized the abilities of that medical treatment which is found efficacious for a particular illness. They have considered their own previous experiences while selecting one mode of medical treatment. Gould opined : "a kind of folk pragmatism acts as a selective principle to help determine which method of treatment is to be chosen" (1957:515).

While evaluating the overall effect of modern medicine upon the tribal community in general and ethnomedicine in particular, one can find that instead of competition or contradiction, there exists an atmosphere of coexistence and division of labour. The tribals employ their own pragmatism to decide what type of medicine must be used for a particular illness and use it accordingly. They resort to both ethnomedicine and modern medicine according to the etiology and seriousness of different illnesses. So, there is ample scope for the survival of both systems of medicine in the tribal universe. Each one deals with the type of disease for which it is found more efficacious. So, in the present circumstances both ethno and modern medical systems play a combined role in the health care of the tribals.

ACCEPTANCE OF MODERN MEDICINE-A CAUTIONARY NOTE

In the present age one may be tempted to presume that modern medicine has taken over ethnomedicine and is the sole agent of health care for the tribals. But such an assumption would be much far from the reality. The acceptance of modern medicine does not mean that people have lost all their faith in the ethnomedical system. Rather they choose different types of medicines for various illnesses according to the advantages of each one of them. So the old practices exist along with the new innovations. Nichter has observed: "the acceptance of modern medicine has not meant that traditional ideas of disease etiology have been superseded or that the cultural ramifications of specific illness have disappeared" (1981:224). Bhardwaj (1985) and Bhat (1976) have also reached similar conclusions from their studies.

The tribals have a number of definite patterns of selection related to various sociocultural factors while deciding to avail any of the medical systems. Nichter (op. cit., p. 225) has explained: "these patterns of resort are dependent on multiple factors including economic and educational variables, the influence of local practitioners, the cultural significance of an illness and the strategic use of illness as a means of role manipulation and/or expression of anxiety."

For chronic illnesses like rheumatism and supernatural diseases like evil eye the tribals show preference to use ethnomedicine, while for other types of diseases originated from natural causes people prefer modern medicine. The division of diseases for the two systems of medicine is not distinct and is much subjective in nature. Gould found that "the villagers were pragmatists who resort to whatever systems of medicine were available and seemed valuable to them". (1965:201).

COOPERATION BETWEEN MODERN AND ETHNOMEDICINE

Modern medicine has come to stay among the tribes and it flourishes along with ethnomedicine which is still strong in the tribal universe. Both play relevant roles in their health care and the tribals exploit the facilities of the two systems with a sense of pragmatism. As the ultimate aim of both systems of medicine is to preserve the health of people by fighting against diseases, integration of modern medicine in the health care system of the tribals would be beneficial to the health of the tribal community. Total displacement of ethnomedicine will not be feasible at this stage and if attempted will be fatal to the tribals. In the ethnomedicine, there are certain components which could be retained because of their ecological and environmental advantages. Integration of modern medicine with the health habits of the tribals may appear simple and easily achievable but a number of ideological and practical hurdles are present in the way of attaining this goal.

The attitude of both doctors and medicinemen has to be changed for attaining cooperation between these two systems of medicine. At present they have no common ground for meeting. Each looks at the other with suspicion. The modern physician, additionally, has contempt for ethnomedicine and this makes the tribals more suspicious of the doctors. A better understanding of each other's domains through successful communication is essential for the development of such a friendly atmosphere.

It is a common complaint of the health administrators that the tribals are not cooperating with them whenever they implement medical programmes for their benefit. But the administrators do not realize that this problem is arising due to. the lack of understanding about this new medical system. So, imparting awareness among the tribals about modern medicine, is an essential step for carrying out the medical programmes successfully.

New avenues must be opened to bring forth chances of better cooperation between the personnel of both systems of medicine. Such an understanding will be more useful for a modern medical practitioner. Then only he can interpret the behaviour of the tribal patients and understand why they are responding in a particular fashion on certain occasions. After getting a clear knowledge of their concepts of disease etiology and healing, he can behave towards them in a better and more acceptable manner. "Before attempting to work for a people we have to learn all about their way of life and why they do what they do" (Ramunny, 1987:3).

On the other hand the tribal medicinemen also can be made aware of the importance and necessity of personal hygiene, safe drinking water, home sanitation and environmental sanitation. The medicinemen can easily grasp these ideas as they possess a rudimentary knowledge about health and healing . Through proper methods of health education these ideas can be broadened and their doubts can be cleared. The cooperation and assistance of the medicinemen are crucial for the successful implementation of health programmes in tribal communities.

HEALTH EDUCATION : THE URGENT NEED

Besides enlightening the tribal medicinemen about various aspects of health care, the community as a whole needs to be made aware of this subject through adequate programmes of health education. A general awakening of the community for the betterment of their living conditions has to be generated by executing these programmes. At present, the necessity and importance of health education for uplifting the standard of health of the tribals and other rural masses is generally accepted in the country. "Health education should be an essential component of all health care; and the health care services should assume special responsibility for the health education of the poor and underprivileged groups who need it most (ICSSR-ICMR, 1981).

So, suitable programmes must be chalked out and implemented with the cooperation of the community as a whole and the medicinemen in particular for educating the tribals about the basic necessities of health care like preservation of safe drinking water, personal hygiene, home sanitation, environmental sanitation, prevention of the spreading of epidemics etc. Education can also be imparted on preventive measures like immunisation programmes and about family welfare programmes.

Low cost latrines have to be constructed for the sanitary disposal of waste and water supply schemes also should be implemented for providing safe drinking water in the tribal areas. Then the people have to be educated about the necessity for improvement of personal hygiene, sanitary disposal of waste and the economical use of drinking water, in a manner that will improve individual and community health. The participation of the people in the implementation and management of these community health schemes would be of crucial importance, both for reducing the costs of their construction as well as to see that the beneficiaries value and protect the services provided to them.

The tribal people can be advised to retain the positive aspects of their ethnomedicine. This traditional mode of health care has proved its versatility and efficiency by preserving the health of people for centuries. While introducing the modern ways of health care, special efforts must be made to enlighten them about the utility of their ethnomedicine. The knowledge of the tribals about their indigenous medicines can play an important role in strengthening modern primary health care. They are economical and culturally accepted programmes of community health care.

So, the health educators must have a sufficient knowledge of the concepts of health and disease in the community in which they are going to work. This will help them to make appropriate suggestions which are suitable for the cultural background of that particular community. Then only the beneficiaries will accept the programmes planned for them, without any hesitation. Maclean has opined : "Health education in its widest sense will not begin to be effective without a prior understanding of the medical philosophy which it is presuming to replace" (1966:139).

CONCLUSION

This study has succeeded in shedding light on certain unexplored aspects of tribal culture. An analysis of the empirical data collected during this investigation really proved certain points beyond and doubts. Such information are also valuable in developing appropriate health care programmes for tribal communities. Like any other investigation this study also may raise many new questions in the mind of a reader. The major findings can be summarized as follows :

The ethnomedicine of tribals is in a process of change due to the interaction with other clusters. Initially, the non-tribal immigrants from the plains influenced the tribal culture in a big way. Afterwards, the introduction of modern medicine into the tribal universe by both governmental and private agencies affected ethnomedicine and brought changes into this system. However, the nature of interaction between modern and ethnomedicine and the subsequent social change among various tribal communities are not similar everywhere.

Even in this transitional period, considerable number of ethnomedical beliefs and practices are still persisting in the tribal communities. It is evident that, in the concepts of etiology, in the treatment of diseases and in the prophylactic measures the traditional medical beliefs and practices are still prevailing. It is also noticed that the various elements of ethnomedicine are reinforced by the principles of tribal religion.

Tribals take to modern medicine only when the illness is an imported one or one which cannot be explained in terms of tribal logic. It is understood that the tribals possess effective methods in their ethnomedicine to treat the diseases which are present among them since the remote past. However, they do not know how to heal the newly imported diseases and, therefore, seek the assistance of modern medicine.

The confrontation between ethnomedicine and modern medicine resulted in a co-existence of the two and a division of labour. The introduction of modern medicine did not result in the complete destruction of ethnomedicine. Depending upon the nature of disease etiology and mode of treatment the tribals pragmatically avail the services of both systems.

Bibliography

Ahluwalia, Aneeta. 1974. "Sociology of Medicine", in M. N. Srinivas et. al. (ed) *A Survey of Research in Sociology and Social Anthropology*, Vol.-II. Bombay : Popular Prakashan.

Aiyappan, A. 1937. "Social and Physical Anthropology of the Nayadis of Malabar". *Bulletin of the Madras Government Museum, General Section*, Vol.2, No. 4.

Aiyappan, A. 1965. *Social Revolution in a Kerala Village*. Bombay : Asia Publishing House.

Ali, Almas. 1987. "Tribal Health Research : Issues and Challenges." Paper presented at the National Workshop on Tribal Health and Medicine in Forest Environment. Dept. of KIRTADS, Kozhikode, Kerala.

Anonymous. 1972. "The Problem of Health and Medical Service in Tribal Areas". *Hill India*, Vol. 1, No.2.

Antia, N. H. 1985.. "An Alternative Strategy for Health Care. The Mandwa Project." *Economic and Political Weekly*, Vol. XX, Nos. 51 and 52.

Atkinson, Jane Monnig. 1987. "The Effectiveness of Shamans in an Indonesian Ritual." *American Anthropologist,* Vol. 89, No.2.

Balzer, Mandelstam Marjorie. 1983. "Doctors or Deceivers? The Siberian Khanty Shaman and Soviet Medicine", in Lola, Romanucci-Ross et. al. (ed.) *The Anthropology of Medicine,* Massachusetts: Bergin and Garvey Publishers Inc.

Banerji, Debabar. 1989. "Class Inequalities and unequal Access to Health Services in India". *Social Action,* Vol-39, No.3.

Banerji, Debabar. 1989. "Rural Social Transformation and changes in Health Behaviour". *Economic and Political Weekly,* Vol.XXIV, No.26.

Beals, Allan R. et. al. 1973. *Culture in Process.* Newyork: Holt, Rinehart and Winston Inc.

Beals, Ralph L. et. al. 1977. *An Introduction to Anthropology.* Newyork: Macmillan Publishing Company.

Beattie, John. 1964. *Other Cultures.* Newyork : The Free Press.

Bellah, Robert N. 1968. "The Sociology of Religion", in Talcott Parsons (ed) *American Sociology : Perspectives, Problems, Methods. Newyork* : Basic Books Inc.

Betteille, Andre. 1977. "The Definition of Tribe" in Romesh Thaper (ed.) *Tribe, Caste and Religion in India.* Delhi: The Macmillan Company.

Bhardwaj, M. 1985. "Attitude Towards different systems of Medicine—A Survey of Four

Villages in Punjab," in Akhtar Rais and Learmonth, A.T.A (eds.) *Geographical aspects of Health and Disease in India. New Delhi* : Concept Publishing Company.

Bhat, K.H. 1976. "Medicinemen of Basavanhalli : A Study of Ethnomedicine". *Journal of the Indian Anthropological Society*, Vol.II, No.1.

Bhattacharya. 1975. *Ancient Indian Rituals and their Social Contents.* Delhi : Manohar Book Service.

Bhattacharya, S. and Sengupta, Syamal Kanti. 1986. "The Concept of Disease and its Treatment among the Birhors of Purulia", in Buddhadeb Chaudhuri (ed.) *Tribal Health.* New Delhi: Inter India Publications.

Bhowmick, K.L. and Chowdhury, J Basuroy. 1976. "Sociocultural Barriers to Technological Change : An Anthropological Approach", in Francis X. Grollig and Harold B. Haley (eds.) *Medical Anthropology*. The Hague : Mouton Publishers.

Bhowmick, P.K. and Bagchi, Tilak. 1987. "Sociocultural and Environmental Factors of Health". Paper presented at the National Workshop on Tribal Health and Medicine in Forest Environment. Dept. of KIRTADS-Kozhikode, Kerala.

Bose, Ashish and Desai, P.B. 1983. *Studies in Social Dynamics of Primary Health Care.* Delhi : Hindustan Publishing Corporation.

Brown, A.R. Radcliffe. 1976. *Structure and Function in Primitive Society.* London : Routledge and Kegan Paul Ltd.

Brown, Ina Corinne. 1963. *Understanding Other Cultures*. New Jersy: Prentice-Hall Inc.

Burton, John W. 1985. "Why Witches? Some Comments on the Explanation of Illusions in Anthropology". *Ethnology*, Vol. XXIV, No. 4

Carstairs, G Morris : 1955. "Medicine and Faith in Rural Rajasthan, " In B.D. Paul (ed.) *Health, Culture and Community*. Newyork: Russell Sage Foundation.

Carstairs, G Morris. 1983. *Death of a Witch*. London: Hutchinson and Co. Ltd.

Census of India, 1981. "Primary Census Abstract for Scheduled Castes and Scheduled Tribes." Director of Census Operations, Kerala.

Chakraborty, Aniruddha. 1986. "Some Findings on the use of Traditional Medicine in the Rural Areas of Palamau", in Buddhadeb Chaudhuri (ed.), *Tribal Health*. New Delhi : Inter-India Publications.

Chaudhuri, Buddhadeb. 1989. "Social Sciences, Health and Culture : The Tribal Situation." *Social Action*, Vol.39, No.3

Chilivumbo, A.B. 1976. "Social Basis of Illness : A Search for Therapeutic Meaning", in Francis X. Grollig and Harold B. Haley (eds.) *Medical Anthropology*. The Hague : Mouton Publishers.

Chowdhuri, M.K. et. al. 1986. "Impact of Prevalent Diseases among the Tribals of Tribal concentrated Areas of West Bengal", in Buddhadeb Chaudhuri (ed.) *Tribal Health*. New Delhi : Inter-India Publications.

Clune, Jr. Francis J. 1976. "Witchcraft, The Shaman and Active Pharmacopoeia", in Francis X. Grollig and Harold B. Haley (eds.) *Medical Anthropology*. The Hague : Mouton Publishers.

Cockburn, Aidan. 1977. "Where did Our Infectious Diseases come from ? The Evolution of Infectious Diseases", in *Health and Disease in Tribal Societies*. C I B A Foundation Symposium 49. New York: Elsevier-Excerpta Medica.

Das, T. C. 1963. "Aspects of Tribal Culture under modern impact in Eastern India", in Bala Ratnam (ed.) *Anthropology On the March*. Madras : Social Sciences Association.

Dash, Jagannath. 1986. "The Concept and Treatment of Disease in Tribal Orissa" in Buddhadeb Chaudhuri (ed.) *Tribal Health*. New Delhi: Inter India Publications.

Desai, A.R. 1977. "Tribes in Transition", in Romesh Thaper (ed.) *Tribe, Caste and Religion in India*. Delhi : The Macmillan Company.

Dhebar, U.N. 1961. "Report of the Scheduled Areas and Scheduled Tribes Commission", Vol.I . Delhi : Government of India Press.

Djurfeldt, Goran and Lindberg, Staffan. 1976. *Pills Against Poverty-A Study of the Introduction of Western Medicine in a Tamil Village*. New Delhi : Oxford and IBH Publishing Company.

Dubois, Abbe J.A. 1981. *Hindu Manners, Customs and Ceremonies*. Delhi : Oxford University Press.

Egnor, Margaret Trawick. 1984. "The Changed Mother or what Smallpox Goddess did when there was no more Smallpox", in E.V. Daniel and J.F. Pugh (eds.), *Contributions to Asian Studies*, Vol-18. The Netherlands : E.J. Brill, Leiden.

Ehrenfels, U. R. 1952. *Kadars of Cochin*. Madras : University of Madras.

Elwin, Verrier. 1955. *The Religion of an Indian Tribe*. London : Oxford University Press.

Etkin, Nina L. and Ross, Paul J. 1983. "Malaria, Medicine and Meals : Plant use among the Hausa and its impact on Disease", in L.R. Ross et. al (ed.) *The Anthropology of Medicine*. Massachusetts: Bergin and Garvey Publishers Inc.

Fabrega, Jr. Horacio. 1972. "Medical Anthropology", in B.J. Siegal (ed). *Biennial Review of Anthropology*. Stanford, California : Stanford University Press.

Fabrega, Jr. Horacio and Manning, Peter K. 1972. "Health Maintenance among Peruvian Peasants". *Human Organization*, Vol. 31, No.3.

Fejos, Paul. 1968. "Magic, Witchcraft and Medical Theory in Primitive Cultures" in Alan Dundes (ed.) *Every Man His Way-Readings in Cultural Anthropology*. New Jersey : Prentice-Hall Inc.

Felson, Richard B and Gmelch, George. 1979. "Uncertainty and the use of Magic". *Current Anthropology*, Vol.20, No.3.

Finkler, Kaja. 1983. "Studying Outcomes of Mexican Spiritualist Therapy", in L.R. Ross et.al. (ed.) *The Anthropology of Medicine.* Massachusetts : Bergin and Garvey Publishers Inc.

Firth, Raymond. 1971. *Elements of Social Organization.* London: Tavistock Publications.

Fortes, Meyer. 1961. *"Mind".* in E.E.Evans Pritchard (ed.) *The Institutions of Primitive Society.* Oxford: Basil, Blackwell and Mott Ltd.

Foster, George M. 1962. *Traditional Cultures and the impact of Technological Change.* New York : Harper and Row Publishers.

Foster, George M. 1965. "Peasant Society and the Image of Limited Good" *American Anthropologist,* Vol.67, No.2.

Foster, George M. 1976. "Disease Etiologies in Non-Western Medical Systems". *American Anthropologist,* Vol.78, No. 4

Fuchs, Stephen. 1949. *The Children of Hari. Ahemadabad* : The New Order Book Company.

Fuchs, Stephen. 1973. *The Aboriginal Tribes of India.* Delhi: The Macmillan Company.

Gallus, A. 1972. "A Bio functional Theory of Religion". *Current Anthropology,* Vol.13, No.5.

Ghosh, J.N. 1960. "Health Measures in NEFA", in *The Adivasis.* New Delhi : Director Publications Division, Government of India.

Glaser, William A. 1968. "Medical Care-Social Aspects", in David L. Sills (ed.) *International Encyclopaedia of Social Sciences,* Vol.10. New York : The Macmillan and Free Press.

Glick, Leonard B. 1967. "Medicine as an Ethnographic Category : The Gimi of the New Guinea Highlands". *Ethnology*, Vol.VI, No.l.

Gnanambal, K. 1955. "The Religious Beliefs of the Urali". *Bulletin of the Department of Anthropology*, Vol. IV, No.2.

Gonzalez, Nancie Solien. 1966. "Health Behaviour in Cross-Cultural Perspective : A Guatemalan Example". *Human Organization*, Vol.25, No.2.

Gorer, Geoffrey. 1967. *Himalayan Village-An account of the Lepchas of Sikkim*. London : Thomas Nelson and Sons Ltd.

Gould, H.A.1957. "The Implications of Technological change for Folk and Scientific Medicine". *American Anthropologist*, Vol.59, No.3.

Gould, H.A. 1965. "Modern Medicine and Folk Cognition in Rural India". *Human Organization*, Vol.24, No.3

Graburn, H.H.Nelson and Strong, B.S. 1973. *Circumpolar Peoples : An Anthropological Perspective*. California : Good Year Publishing Company.

Grottanelli, Vingi L. 1976. "Witchcraft : An Allegory" in Francis X. Grollig and Harold B. Haley (eds.) *Medical Anthropology*. The Hague : Mouton Publishers.

Guha, Anima. 1986. "Folk Medicine of the Boro-Kacharis-A Plains Tribe of Assam", in Buddhadeb Chaudhuri (ed.), *Tribal Health*. New Delhi : Inter-India Publications.

Gupta, Beni. 1979. *Magical Beliefs and Superstitions.* Delhi : Sundeep Prakashan.

Gupta, P.N. Sen and Biswas, S.K. 1956. "Studies on the Diet and Nutritional status of the Malapantaram, Muthuvan and Ullatan Tribes of Travancore". *Bulletin of the Department of Anthropology,* Vol.V, No.2.

Gupta, P.D. 1984. *Life and culture of a Matrilineal Tribe of Meghalaya.* New Delhi : Inter India Publications.

Hahn, Robert A. 1984. "Rethinking Illness and Disease", in E.V. Daniel and J.F. Pugh (ed.) *Contributions to Asian Studies,* Vol.18. The Netherlands : E.J. Brill, Leiden.

Harris, Marvin. 1983. *Cultural Anthropology.* New York : Harper and Row Publishers.

Hasan, K.A. 1967. *The Cultural Frontier of Health in Village India.* Bombay : Manaktala and Sons Pvt. Ltd.

Hasanin, Nadeem. 1983. *Tribal India Today.* New Delhi: Harnam Publications.

Henry, Edward O. 1981. "A North-Indian Healer and the Sources of his Power, " in Giri Raj Gupta (ed) *Main Currents in Indian Sociology,* Vol.IV. New Delhi : Vikas.

Herrick, James W. 1983. "The Symbolic Roots of three potent Iroquois Medicinal Plants", in L.R. Ross et. al. (ed) *The Anthropology of Medicine.* Massachusetts : Bergin and Garvey Publishers Inc.

Herskovits, Melville J. 1955. *Cultural Anthropology.* New Delhi : Oxford and IBH Publishing Company.

Herzfeld, Michael. 1986. "Closure as Cure : Tropes in the Exploration of Bodily and Social Disorder." *Current Anthropology,* Vol.27, No.2.

Hockings, Paul. 1980. *Sex and Disease in a Mountain Community.* New Delhi : Vikas.

Hoebel, E. Adamson. 1958. *Man in the Primitive World-An Introduction to Anthropology.* New York : Mc Graw and Hill Book Company Inc.

Hoff, Wilbur and Maseko, D. Nhlavana. 1986. "Nurses and 'Traditional. Healers Join Hands." *World Health Forum,* Vol.7, No. 4.

Howells, William. 1956. *Man in the Beginning, The Story of Our own Origins . London :* G. Bell and Sons Ltd.

Hughes, Charles C. 1968. "Medical Care-Ethnomedicine", in David L. Sills (ed.) *International Encyclopedia of the Social Sciences,* Vol. 10. New York : The Macmillan Co. and The Free Press.

ICSSR-ICMR. 1980. "Health for All, An Alternative Strategy" *I C S S R Newsletter* Vol. XI (1).

Iyer, L.A. Krishna. 1937. *The Travancore Tribes and Castes,* Vol.I Trivandrum : Government Press.

Iyer, L.A. Krishna. 1939. *The Travancore Tribes and Castes,* Vol.II. Trivandrum : Government Press.

Iyer, L.A. Krishna. 1941. *The Travancore Tribes and Castes,* Vol.III. Trivandrum : Government Press.

Iyer, L. A. Krishna. 1961. *Kerala and Her People.* Palghat : The Educational Supplies Dept.

Iyer, L.K. Anantha Krishna. 1908. *Cochin Tribes and Castes.* Cochin : Higginbotham and Company.

Jaggi, O.P. 1980. *History of Science, Technology and Medicine in India,* Vol. XV.Delhi : Atma Ram and Sons.

Jain, S.K. (ed.), 1981. *Glimpses of Indian Ethnobotany.* New Delhi : Oxford and I BH Publishing Company.

Johnson, Allen W. 1978. *Research Methods In Social Anthropology.* London : Edward Arnold Ltd.

Jones, Delmos J. 1970. "Towards a Native Anthropology." *Human Organization,* Vol.29, No. 4.

Jones, David A. 1977. "Medical Practice and Tribal Communities", in *Health and Disease in Tribal Societies.* CIBA Foundation Symposium 49. New York : Elsevier Excerpta Medica.

Joseph, A. N. T. 1989. "Ethnozoology of Reptiles in Relation to Health Care among Tribals in Madhya Pradesh." *Social Action,* Vol.39, No. 4.

Kakar, D. N. 1977. *Folk and Modern Medicine.* Delhi : New Asian Publishers.

Karna, M. N. 1976. "Etiology of Disease : A Sociological study in the Rural Context." Man in India, Vol. 56, No.1

Kattakayam, Jacob John. 1983. *Social Structure and Change Among the Tribals.* Delhi : D. K. Publications.

Kennedy, John G. 1967. "Nubian Zar Ceremonies as Psychotherapy." *Human Organization*, Vol.26, No. 4.

Khare, R. S. 1959. "A Plea for Cultural Dimension in Medicine." *The Eastern Anthropologist*, Vol.12, No.3.

Khare, R. S. 1981. "Folk Medicine in a North Indian Village : Some further Notes and Observations, " in Giri Rai Gupta (ed.) *Main Currents in Indian Sociology*, Vol.IV. New Delhi : Vikas.

Kiev, Ari. 1966. "Obstacles to Medical Progress in Haiti." *Human Organization*, Vol.25, No.1

Kiteme, Kamuti. 1976. "Traditional African Medicine, " in Francis X. Grollig and Harold B. Haley (eds.) *Medical Anthropology*. The Hague : Mouton Publishers.

Lewis, G. A. 1977. "Beliefs and Behaviour in Disease", in *Health and Disease in Tribal Societies*. C I B A Foundation Symposium 49. New York : Elsevier-Excerpta-Medica.

Lewis, Walter H and Elwin, Lewis. 1977. *Medical Botany-Plants affecting Man's Health*. New York : John Wiley and Sons Inc.

Lieban, Richard W. 1973. "Medical Anthropology", in John J. Honigman (ed.) *Handbook of Social and cultural Anthropology*. Chicago : Rand Mc Nally College Publishing Company.

Luiz, A. A. D. 1962. *Tribes of Kerala*. New Delhi : Bharatiya Adimjati Sevak Sangh.

Maclean, Catherine M.U. 1966. "Hospitals or Healers ? An attitude Survey in Ibadan." *Human Organization*, Vol.25, No.2.

Madan, T.N. 1969. "Who Chooses Modern Medicine and Why. "*Economic and 'olitical Weekly*, Vol.4, No.37.

Mahapatra, Sitakant. 1986. *Modernization and Ritual : Identity and Change in Santal Society*. Calcutta : Oxford University Press.

Majumdar, D.N. 1961. *Races and cultures of India*. Bombay: Asia Publishing House.

Majumdar, D.N. 1968. 'An Account of Magico-Religious Rites and Beliefs of the Rongdani Rabha." *Bulletin Of the Anthropological Survey of India*, Vol-XVII, No. 3.

Majumdar, D.N. 1984. "Approach to Tribal Problems, " in L.P. Vidyarthi (ed.) *Applied Anthropology, India*. Allahabad : Kitab Mahal.

Mandelbaum, David G. 1970. "Curing and Religion in South Asia." *Journal of Indian Anthropological Society*, Vol. V, Nos.1 and 2.

Mandelbaum, David G. 1981. "Transnatural Curing," in Giri Raj Gupta (ed.) *Main Currents in Indian Sociology*, Vol. IV. New Delhi : Vikas Publishing House.

Mani, S.B. 1981. "From Marriage to child conception : an Ethnomedical Survey in rural Tamilnadu, " in Giri Raj Gupta (ed.) *Main Currents in Indian Sociology*, Vol.IV. New Delhi : Vikas Publishing House.

Mankad, Dhruv. 1987. "Health under Capitalism." *Economic and Political Weekly*, Vol. XXII, No.5

Mann, R.S. 1979. *Social Structure, Social Change*

and Future Trends. Jaipur Rawat Publications.

Maquet, Jacques J. 1964. "Objectivity in Anthropology.' *Current Anthropology*, Vol. 20, No.1.

Marriott, Mc Kim. 1955. "Western Medicine in a village of Northern India, " in B. D. Paul (ed.) *Health, Culture and Community*. New York : Russell Sage Foundation.

Mathur, P.R.G. 1977. *Tribal Situation in Kerala.* Trivandrum : Kerala Historical Society.

Mathur, P.R.G. 1982. "Anthropology of Tribal Medicine : Disease and Curing Techniques among the Tribals of North Wynad (Kerala)". *Man in India*, Vol.62, No.3.

Mathur, P.R.G. 1987. "The Ethnomedicine of the Irular of Attapady, Kerala." Paper presented at the National Workshop on Anthropology of Tribal Health and Medicine in Forest Environment. Dept. of KIRTADS, Kozhikode, Kerala.

Matthews, C.M.E. 1978. "Health and Village Culture in Tamilnadu.' *Social Action*, Vol.28, No.3.

Matthews, C.M.E. 1979. *Health and Culture in a South Indian Village*. New Delhi : Sterling Publishers.

Menon, Ramesh. 1988. "The Influence of Spirits". *India Today*, Vol.XIII, No.22.

Micozzi, Marc S. 1983. "Anthropological Study of Health Beliefs, Behaviours and outcomes : Traditional Folk Medicine and

Ethnopharmacology.' *Human Organization*, Vol.42, No.4.

Mishra, Narayan. 1978. *Cultural Persistence and Change-A Rural Profile of Anjan.* New Delhi : Classical Publications.

Moerman, Daniel E. 1979 "Anthropology of Symbolic Healing." *Current Anthropology*, Vol.20. No.1.

Mishra, P.K. 1985. "Ecological Stability in Tribal Lifestyles," in J. Bandyopadhyay et al. (eds) *India's Environment : Crises and Responses.* Dehra Dun : Natraj Publishers.

Mohandas, K. 1987. "Culture change and Physical Characteristics of Paliyans of Kerala." Unpublished Ph.D Thesis submitted to University of Kerala, Thiruvananthapuram.

Moorthy, O.K. 1972. "The Tribal Situation in South India, " in Suresh K. Sing (ed.) *The Tribal situation in India.* Shimla : Indian Institute of Advanced Study.

Mukherjee, B.M. 1986. "Aging Members and their Health in Changing Techno-Economic Condition, " in Buddhadeb Chaudhuri (ed.) *Tribal Health.* New Delhi : Inter-India Publications.

Murdock, George P.1978. "World Distribution Theories of Illness". *Ethnology*, Vol.XVII, No.4.

Myerhoff, B.G. and Larson, W.R. 1965. "The Doctor as Culture Hero : The Routinization of Charisma." *Human Organization*, Vol.24, No.3.

Nagaswami, R. 1980. *Art and Culture of*

Tamilnadu. Delhi : Sundeep Prakashan.

Naik, T.B. 1972. "Applied Anthropology in India, " in M.N. Srinivas et. al. (eds.) *A Survey of Research in Sociology and Social Anthropology.* Bombay : Popular Prakashan.

Naik, T.B. 1984. "What is a Tribe : Conflicting Deflicting, " in L.P. Vidyarthi (ed.) *Applied Anthropology in India.* Allahabad : Kitab Mahal.

Nair, N. Vishwanathan. 1985. "Tribal Health and Medicine in Kerala" Unpublished Ph.D. Thesis submitted to the Calicut University, Kerala.

Nair, N. Vishwanathan. 1987. "Tribes, Healers, Medicinal matter and Environment." Paper presented at the National Workshop on Tribal Health and Medicine in Forest Environment. Dept. of KIRTADS, Kozhikode, Kerala.

Nambiar, V.P.Krishnan et. al. 1985. *Studies on the Medicinal Plants of Kerala Forests.* Peechi : Kerala Forest Research Institute.

Narayan, Ravi. 1989. "Towards a People-Oriented Alternative health care System." *Social Action,* Vol.39, No.3.

Nash, June. 1967. "The logic of Behaviour : Curing in a Maya Indian Town". *Human Organization,* Vol.26, No.3.

Ndeti, Kivuto. 1976. "The Relevance of African Traditional medicine in Modern Medical Training and Practice, " in Francis X. Grollig and Harold B. Haley (eds) *Medical Anthropology.* The Hague : Mouton.

Nehru, Jawaharlal. 1960. "The Tribal Folk, " in *The Adivasis.* New Delhi: Director,

Publications Division, Government of India.

Nichter, Mark. 1981. "Towards a Cultural Responsive Rural Health Care Delivery System in India, " in Giri Raj Gupta (ed.) *Main Currents in Indian Sociology*, Vol. IV. New Delhi: Vikas Publishing House.

Noll, Richard. 1985. Mental Imagery Cultivation as a Cultural Phenomenon : The Role of Visions in Shamanism. *Current Anthropology*, Vol.26, No.4.

Nurge, Ethel. 1958. Etiology of Illness in Guinhangdan. *American Anthropologist*, Vol. 60, No.6.

Palgi, Phyllis. 1983. "Mental Health, Traditional beliefs and the Moral Order among Yemenite Jews in Israel," in L.R. Ross et. al. (eds.) *The Anthropology of Medicine*. Massachusetts : Bergin and Garvey Publishers Inc.

Perrin, Michel. 1987. "Shamanistic Symptoms or Symbols? A case of Indetermination." *Anthropos*, 82, 4/6.

Pfifferling, John Henry. 1976. "Medical Anthropology : Mirror for Medicine," in Francis X. Grollig and Harold B. Haley (eds.) *Medical Anthropology*. The Hague : Mouton.

Poitevin, Guy. 1988. "Primary Health Care as a Gender Issue." *Economic and Political Weekly*, Vol.XXIII, No.41.

Polunin, Ivan. 1977. "Some Characteristics of Tribal People, " in *Health and Disease in Tribal Societies*. CIBA Foundation Symposium 49. New York : Elsevier-Excerpta Medica.

Queiroz, S. Marcos. 1984. Hot and Cold Classification in Traditional Iguape Medicine. *Ethnology* Vol.XXIII, No.1

Radhakrishnan, V.N. 1985. "The Traditional Medicine of Kanikkars." *Kalpadhenu* Vol.13, No.3

Rai, Suman. 1988. Impact of Forest Policies on Forest Dwellers. *Social Welfare*, Vol.XXXV, No.8

Ramunny, Murkot. 1987. "Anthropology of Tribal Health and Medicine in Forest Environment- An Administrators Experiences." Paper presented at the National Workshop on Anthropology of Tribal health and Medicine in Forest Environment. Dept. of KIRTADS, Kozhikode, Kerala.

Rao, M.S.A. 1986. Supernatural possession in Kerala. *Man in India*, Vol. 66, No.1

Reddy, Rami V 1987 "Tribal Health : Social-Cultural and Biological." Paper presented at the National Workshop on Anthropology of Tribal Health and Medicine in Forest Environment. Dept. of KIRTADS, Kozhikode, Kerala.

Rogers, S.L. and Evernham Lorraine. 1983. "Shamanistic Healing among the Diegueno Indians of Southern California, " in L.R. Ross et. al. (eds.) *Anthropology of Medicine*. Massachusetts : Bergin and Garvey Publishers Inc.

Rizvi, S.N.H. 1986. "Health Practices of the Jaunsaries - A Socio- Cultural Analysis, " in Budhadeb Chaudhuri (ed) *Tribal Health*. New

Delhi : Inter-India Publications.

Romesh Thaper (ed.). 1977. *Tribe, Caste and Religion in India.* New Delhi : The Macmillan Company.

Rosengren, William R.1980. *Sociology of Medicine : Diversity, Conflict and Change.* New York : Harper and Row Publishers.

Sahu, S.K. 1987. "Health of the Tribes Issues and Perspectives." Paper presented at the National Workshop on Tribal Health and Medicine in Forest Environment. Dept. of KIRTADS, Kozhikode, Kerala.

Saksena, R.N. 1978. "The Tribes of India", in Ratish Srivastava (ed.) *Social Anthropology in India. New Delhi:* Oriental Publishers.

Saraswati, Baidyanath. 1987. "Tribal Ayurveda Must we destroy it." Paper presented at the National Workshop on Tribal Health and Medicine in Forest Environment. Dept. of KIRTADS, Kozhikode, Kerala.

Saunders, Lyle. 1954. "Healing Ways" in J.D.Jennings and E.A. Hoebel (eds.) *Readings in Anthropology.* New York : MC Graw-Hill Book Company.

Sengupta, Syamalkanti. 1977. *Applied Anthropology : Meaning and necessity.* Calcutta: Firm K L M Private Ltd.

Sen, Tulika. 1986. "The Health-Status of the Residual Andamanese," in Buddhadeb Chaudhuri (ed.) *Tribal Health.* New Delhi Inter India Publications.

Shankar, Darshan. 1985. "Cultural Cross-Current-Tribal Medicine, Ayurveda and Modern Medicine, in the context of Primary Health

Care". *Ancient Science of life,* Vol.V, No.2.

Sharma, Monica. 1984. "Health Profile of India-Problems, Services and Issues". *Journal of the Indian Anthropological Society,* Vol.19, No.2.

Shiloh, Ailon. 1965. "A Case Study of Disease and Culture in Action: Leprosy Among the Hausa of Northern Nigeria." *Human Organization,* Vol.24, No.2.

Sigerist, Henry E. 1943. *Civilization and Disease.* Chicago The University of Chicago : Press.

Simmons, Ozzie G. 1960. "Popular and Modern Medicine in Mestizo Communities, " in Dorrian Apple (ed) *Sociological Studies on Health and Sickness.* New York : Mc Graw-Hill Book Company, Inc.

Singh, Ajit K. 1984. *Tribal Development in India.* Delhi : Amar Prakashan.

Singh, Amar Kumar. 1984. "Health Modernity : Concepts and Correlates." *Social Change,* Vol.14, No.3.

Spradly, James P and Mc Curdy, David W. 1980. *Anthropology - The Cultural Perspective.* New York : John Wiley and Sons, Inc.

Statement on National Health Policy :1982. New Delhi Ministry of Health and Family Welfare, Government of India.

Thomas, P.T. 1963. "Adjustments to Changing Environment," in Bala Ratnam (ed.) *Anthropology on the March.* Madras : Social Sciences Association.

Thurston, Edgar. 1907. *Ethnographic Notes in Southern India.* Delhi : Cosmo Publications.

Thurston, Edgar. 1909. *Castes and Tribes of Southern India.* Delhi : Cosmo Publications.

Tiwari, S.C. 1987. "Health and Disease in the Tribes of Uttara Khand." Paper presented at the National Workshop on Tribal Health and Medicine in Forest Environment. Dept. of KIRTADS, Kozhikode, Kerala.

Troisi, J. 1979. *Tribal Religion : Religious Beliefs and Practices among the Santals.* New Delhi : Manohar Publications.

Upadhyay, V.S. 1987. "Health in Forest Environment." Paper presented at the National Workshop on Tribal Health and Medicine in Forest Environment. Dept. of KIRTADS, Kozhikode, Kerala.

Van Der Veen, Klass W. 1981. "Sociocultural aspects of Medical Care in Valsad District, Gujarat State, " in Giri Raja Gupta (ed.) *Main Currents in Indian Sociology,* Vol.IV. New Delhi Vikas Publishing House.

Vidyarthi, L.P and Rai, B.K. 1977. *Tribal Culture in India.* Delhi : Concept Publishing Company.

Vidhyarthi, L.P. 1978. *Rise of Anthropology in India,* Vol.I. *The Tribal Dimensions.* Delhi : Concept Publishing Company.

Vidyarthi, L.P. 1984. "History of Applied Anthropology in India, " in self (ed.) *Applied Anthropology in India.* Allahabad : Kitab Mahal.

Vivelo, Frank Robert. 1978. *Cultural Anthropology Handbook.* New York : Mc Graw-Hill Book company.

Wax, Murray, 1968. "Religion and Magic," in James A. Clifton (ed.) *Introduction to Cultural Anthropology*. Boston : Houghton Mifflin Company.

Weaver, Thomas. 1970. "Use of Hypothetical situations in a study of Spanish American Illness Referral Systems". *Human Organization*, Vol.29, No.2.

White, Isobel M. 1977. "Pitfalls to Avoid : The Australian Experience," in *Health and Disease in Tribal Societies*. CIBA Foundation Symposium 49. New York : Elsevier-Excerpta Medica.

Willis, Roy. 1978. "Magic and Medicine in Ufipa, " in Peter Morley and Roy Wallis (eds.) *Culture and Curing*. London : Peter Owen Ltd.

Wirsing, Rolf L. 1985. "The Health of Traditional Societies and the effects of Acculturation." *Current Anthropology*, Vol.26, No.3

Wolff, Robert J. 1965. "Modern Medicine and Traditional Culture : Confrontation on the Malay Peninsula." *Human Organization*, Vol.24, No.4.

Woods, Clyde M and Gravens, T. D. 1976 "The Process of Medical Change in a Highland Guatemalan Town, " in Francis X. Grollig and Harold B. Haley (eds.) *Medical Anthropology*. The Hague : Mouton Publishers.

Young, Allan. 1976. "Some Implications of Medical beliefs and practices for social Anthropology." *American Anthropologist*, Vol.78, No.l.

Index

E

M